Gender, Society & Development

**Gender and health: policy and practice
A global sourcebook**

Gender, Society & Development

Gender and health: policy and practice

A global sourcebook

Anke van der Kwaak and Madeleen Wegelin-Schuringa
Guest Editors

CRITICAL REVIEWS AND ANNOTATED

BIBLIOGRAPHIES SERIES

KIT (Royal Tropical Institute), The Netherlands

Oxfam GB

KIT (Royal Tropical Institute)
KIT Publishers
P.O. Box 95001
1090 HA AMSTERDAM
The Netherlands
Telephone: +31 (0) 20 568 8272
Telefax: +31 (0) 20 568 8286
E-mail: publishers@kit.nl
Website: www.kit.nl

Oxfam Publishing
274 Banbury Road
Oxford OX2 7DZ
United Kingdom
Telephone: +44 (0) 1865 311 311
Telefax: +44 (0) 1865 312 600
E-mail: publish@oxfam.org.uk
Website: www.oxfam.org.uk

© 2006 KIT (Royal Tropical Institute),
Amsterdam

First published by KIT Publishers and
Oxfam GB 2006
Guest editors: Anke van der Kwaak and
Madeleen Wegelin-Schuringa
Series editors: Sarah Cummings, Henk van Dam,
and Minke Valk, KIT (Royal Tropical Institute)
Design: Grafisch Ontwerpbureau Agaatsz BNO,
Meppel
Cover: Ad van Helmond, Amsterdam
Lay-out: Nadamo Bos, KIT Publishers
Printing: High Trade, Zwolle

ISBN 90 6832 734 8 (KIT Publishers edition)
available in the EC excluding UK and Ireland
ISBN 0 85598 571 2 (Oxfam GB edition)
available in the rest of the world
Printed and bound in The Netherlands

*Gender and health: policy and practice. A global
sourcebook*
has been developed by KIT (Royal Tropical Institute)
in The Netherlands. It is co-published with Oxfam
GB to increase dissemination.
The views expressed in documents by named authors
are those of the authors, and not necessarily those of
the publishing organizations.

Oxfam GB is a registered charity no. 202918,
and is a member of Oxfam International.

Other titles in the *Gender, Society & Development*
series:
- *Advancing women's status: women and men
  together?*
  M. de Bruyn (ed.)
- *Gender training. The source book.*
  S. Cummings, H. van Dam and M. Valk (eds.)
- *Women's information services and networks.
  A global source book.*
  S. Cummings, H. van Dam and M. Valk (eds.)
- *Institutionalizing gender equality. Commitment,
  policy and practice. A global source book*
  H. van Dam, A. Khadar and M. Valk (eds.)
- *Gender perspectives on property and inheritance.
  A global source book*
  S. Cummings, H. van Dam, A. Khadar and M. Valk
  (eds.)
- *Natural resources management and gender.
  A global source book*
  S. Cummings, H. van Dam and M. Valk (eds.)
- *Gender, citizenship and governance. A global
  source book*
  S. Cummings, H. van Dam and M. Valk (eds.)
- *Gender and ICTs for development. A global
  sourcebook*
  S. Cummings, H. van Dam and M. Valk (series
  eds.)

Contents

Acknowledgements

A major objective of this publication was to document the experiences of practitioners and experts in the South with respect to gender and health issues. The Series Editors are delighted that it has been possible to realize this objective.

Special thanks go to Anke van der Kwaak and Madeleen Wegelin-Schuringa, Guest Editors of this publication, for sharing their knowledge and experience. We would like to record our warm and deep appreciation of Bertha Simwaka Nhlema, C.K. George, Fiona Samuels, Ireen Makwiza, Lifah Sanudi, Mabel Bianco, Madeleen Wegelin-Schuringa, Miriam Zoll, Patnice Nkhonjera, Ravi Verma, Sally Theobald, Sehin Teferra for their valuable contributions to this book.

We also would like to acknowledge with thanks the support of Nel van Beelen, Ilse Egers, Maitrayee Mukhopadhyay and Korrie de Koning.

Acknowledgements also go to Christine Hayes for her input to the bibliography. We would also like to thank Christine Waslander for her invaluable work in the production of this Series and of this book in particular.

Henk, Sarah and Minke
Series Editors, Gender, Society & Development

Acronyms

ABC	Abstinence, Being faithful, and Condom use
ACORD	Agency for Co-operation and Research in Development
AGI	Alan Guttmacher Institute
AIDS	Acquired immune deficiency syndrome
APDA	Afar Pastoralist Development Association, Ethiopia
AR	Alternative rite
ARSRC	African Regional Sexuality Resources Centre
ARROW	Asian-Pacific Resource & Research Centre for Women
ART	Antiretroviral therapy or antiretroviral treatment
ARV	Antiretrovirals
ASCI	Administrative Staff College of India
BCC	Behaviour change communication
BMZ	Bundesministerium für wirtschafliche Zusammenarbeit und Entwicklung, Germany
CAFS	Centre for African Family Studies
CBOs	Community-based organizations
CEDAW	Convention on the Elimination of All Forms of Discrimination against Women
CHANGE	Center for Health and Gender Equity
CHAM	Christian Health Association of Malawi
CHAZ	Christian Health Association of Zambia
CHE	Community-based health educators
CSIS	Center for Strategic and International Studies, United States
DAW	United Nations Division for the Advancement of Women
DAWN	Development of Alternatives with Women for a New Era
DFID	Department for International Development, United Kingdom
ECOS	Comunicaçao em Sexualidade, Brazil
EmOC	Emergency obstetric care
EU	European Union
EWLA	Ethiopian Women Lawyers Association
FC	Female circumcision
FCI	Family Care International
FEIM	Fundación para Estudio en Investigación de la Mujer, Argentina
FGC	Female genital cutting
FGDs	Focus group discussions
FGM	Female genital mutilation
FHI	Family Health International
FORWARD	Foundation for Women's Health Research and Development
FP	Family planning
FPP	Frontiers Prevention Project, Andhra Pradesh, India

GBA	Gender-based analysis
GCWA	Global Coalition on Women and AIDS
GMS	Gender Management System
GRHF	Global Reproductive Health Forum
GTZ	Deutsche Gesellschaft für Technische Zusammenarbeit (German Technical Co-operation)
GWH	Gender and Women's Health department, World Health Organization
HFWC	Health and Family Welfare Centre
HIPNet	Health Information and Publications Network
HIV	Human immune deficiency virus
HSR	Health sector reform
IANWGE	Inter-Agency Network on Women and Gender Equality, United States
ICAD	Interagency Coalition on AIDS and Development
ICPD	International Conference on Population and Development
ICRH	International Centre for Reproductive Health, Belgium
ICRW	International Center for Research on Women
ICW	International Community of Women Living with HIV/AIDS
IDIs	In-depth interviews
IDS	Institute of Development Studies, United Kingdom
IEC	Information, education and communication
IGH	Institute of Gender and Health, Canada
IGWG	Interagency Gender Working Group
IHS	Institute of Health Systems, Andhra Pradesh, India
ILO	United Nations International Labour Organization
INSP	Instituto Nacional de Salud Pública (National Institute of Public Health), Mexico
INSTRAW	United Nations International Research and Training Institute for the Advancement of Women
INTACT	International Network to Analyze, Communicate and Transform the Campaign against Female Genital Cutting
INTERIGHTS	International Centre for the Legal Protection of Human Rights, United Kingdom
IP	Instituto Promundo, Brazil
IPPF	International Planned Parenthood Federation
IPPF/WHR	International Planned Parenthood Federation/Western Hemisphere Region
IV	Intravenous
IWHC	International Women's Health Coalition
IWHM	International Women's Health Movement
KIT	Koninklijk Instituut voor de Tropen (Royal Tropical Institute), the Netherlands
KMG	Kembatta Mentii Gezzima-Tope, Ethiopia
LACWHN	Latin American and Caribbean Women's Health Network
LHW	Lady Health Worker programme, Pakistan
MaP	Men as Partners project, South Africa
MAP	Monitoring the AIDS Pandemic
MDGs	Millennium Development Goals
MNCH	Maternal, newborn and child health
MVP	Mentors in Violence Protection Strategies, Inc., USA
MYWO	Maendeleo Ya Wanawake Organization
NACO	National AIDS Control Organization, India
NCTPE	National Committee on Traditional Practices in Ethiopia

NGO	Non-governmental organization
NIKK	Nordisk Institutt for kvinne- og kjonnsforskning (Nordic Institute for Women's Studies and Gender Research), Norway
NSO	National Statistical Office, USA
NTP	National TB [Control] Programme, Malawi
OVC RAAAP	Rapid Assessment, Analysis, and Action Planning Initiative on behalf of Orphans and other Vulnerable Children in sub-Saharan Africa
PAHO	Pan American Health Organization
RAP-rule	Rights-based approach, Acceptance of young people's sexuality, and Participation of young people
PATH	Program for Appropriate Technology
PEPFAR	President's Emergency Plan for AIDS Relief, United States
PIWH	Pacific Institute for Women's Health
PLA	Participatory learning and appraisal (tools)
PLWH	People Living With HIV/AIDS
POA	Plan of Action
PRB	Population Reference Bureau
PRSP	Poverty Reduction Strategy Paper
RAINBO	Research, Action, and Information Network for the Bodily Integrity of Women
REACH	Research on Equity and Community Health
REDNAC	National Network of Adolescents and Young People for Sexual and Reproductive Health
RH	Reproductive health
RHAG	Reproductive Health Affinity Group, Ford Foundation, United States
RHO	Reproductive Health Outlook
RTI	Reproductive tract infection
SDC	Swiss Agency for Development and Cooperation
SIDA	Swedish International Development Cooperation Agency
SONASO	Soroti Network of AIDS Service Organizations
SSA	Sub-Saharan Africa
SRH	Sexual and reproductive health
SRHR	Sexual and reproductive health and rights
SRVI	Sexual Violence Research Initiative
STD	Sexually transmitted disease
STI	Sexually transmitted infection
SWAps	Sector wide approaches
TB	Tuberculosis
TDR	Special Programme for Research and Training in Tropical Diseases
TRIZ	Theory of Inventive Problem Solving
UN	United Nations
UNAIDS	Joint United Nations Programme on HIV/AIDS
UNASO	Uganda Network of AIDS Service Organizations
UNDP	United Nations Development Programme
UNESCO	United Nations Educational, Scientific and Cultural Organization
UNF	United Nations Foundation
UNFPA	United Nations Population Fund
UNICEF	United Nations Children Fund
UNIFEM	United Nations Fund for Women

UNRISD	United Nations Research Institute for Social Development
USAID	United States Agency for International Development
VCT	Voluntary counselling and testing
VSO	Voluntary Service Overseas, United Kingdom
WFP	United Nations World Food Programme
WHP	Women's Health Project, South Africa
WHO	World Health Organization
WKC	WHO Kobe Centre, Japan
WRA	Women of reproductive age
WRC	White Ribbon Campaign
WWHR	Women for Women's Human Rights
YWCA	Young Women's Christian Association

gender and health: policy and practice

Anke van der Kwaak and Jashodhara Dasgupta

Introduction: Gender and health

This introduction to the sourcebook 'Gender and health' discusses the international context and recent developments in the broad field of gender and health. Gender and health refers to all gender issues in the field of health, health care, suffering and well-being. Thus, this book not only refers to public health or reproductive health alone but genuine gender and clinical health issues are also presented. In this introduction, gaps and challenges in this field will be discussed. New approaches to gender and health, taking the complex realities into account, are crucial. Moreover, the combination of a gender perspective and a rights' discourse is essential for bringing about change.

The articles in this book all give evidence of the need for contextualization, new approaches and the involvement of civil society. They address the issues that need to be tackled in order to ensure that concrete steps in the direction of gender equity and equality have been taken by the year 2015.

History of ideas: gender as a determinant of health status

The growing strength of the women's movement in the 1960s and 1970s challenged the 'medicalization' of women's bodies and the medical construction of woman's health needs as distinct from women's own experiences and priorities (Boston Women's Health Book Collective 1992). The women's movement questioned the fallacy that males, as doctors or partners, knew better or more about women's bodies than women did. Women articulated felt experiences of mental, physical, reproductive and sexual health needs. Analysing their experiences with reference to the social, political and economic forces that shaped health, women explored the connections between race, class and gender based oppression as they affected the health of women.

As far back as the 19th Century, differences in health status between different social groups have been studied with reference to socioeconomic class differences (Farr 1839). The idea of gender as a determinant of the health of women and men appears a century and a half later in research of the late 1980s and the 1990s (Macintyre 1996; Sen et al 2002) when the debate around inequalities in health expanded beyond socioeconomic class to include race and gender. The concepts of gender and gender analysis evolved from feminist thinking which emphasized the social and cultural nature of many of the differences between men and women, particularly the unequal power and status attributed to female and male roles. This thinking slowly filtered into development debates, including those on health and development (Vlassoff and Moreno 2002).

Between the decades of the 1970s and 1990s, the women's health movement in both developed and developing countries moved ahead (Correa 1994) to establish that women's health was affected by the social context including unequal gender relationships. Gender analysis played an important role in creating the ideal around reproductive health accepted globally at the International Conference on Population and Development (ICPD) in Cairo (Cottingham and Myntti 2002). Articulating their experiences of reproduction, sexuality, health and lack of power, women activists put the principles of reproductive health and rights centre stage, compelling governments to acknowledge that state control of women's reproductive capacities was a violation of women's rights.

This was an effective counter argument to economic and demographic theories which were being used to justify population policies that threatened women's health while simultaneously diverting scarce resources away from basic health care for the poor. The women's health movement collectively identified the larger financial forces that were determining the availability and quality of health care for women. Women questioned the low priority given to preventive care for women's health needs in the context of increasing linkages of the medical system with other profit making businesses. Feminists criticized the attempts of the state and market to control women's bodies, especially their reproductive capacities, through the use of male-dominated science and technology.

Concurrently there was a small but growing body of literature that began to explore gendered dimensions (Mundigo 1995) of men's health: why men engaged in more risk-taking behaviour, used fewer preventive services and had low participation in health care despite significant health concerns and problems. From several studies (Doyal 2000), it appeared that constructing and maintaining a male identity often required the taking of risks that could be seriously hazardous to health.

From the evidence, it emerged that men and women are a product of not only their own biology, but also their social experiences in a stratified society and the gendered roles that they enact (Bird and Rieker 1999). When attempting to understand health related differences between women and men, it is important to analyse the complex ways in which biology and social factors interact since social determinants exacerbate biological vulnerabilities (Sen et al 2002). Krieger (2002), for example, provides 12 useful case studies to demonstrate the spectrum of situations where gender relations and sex-linked biology could affect exposure and health outcomes for women and men.

The gender analysis of differences in the health of women and men had to overcome the general predisposition to attribute every difference to an underlying biological basis. Research legitimized the association of reproductive biology with weakness, often being based on assumptions around biological givens. There has also been a tendency to link women's reproductive biology with mental health, illustrated by the use of the term 'hysteria' where mental disturbance is linked to the uterus. These assumptions were not questioned despite being gendered constructions that sanction social discrimination (Sen et al 2002). Knowledge of the body, health and illness is culturally constructed (Sen et al 2002), and this is most evident in the case of medical knowledge about the health needs of women.

Studies have established that women and men have different health needs and outcomes because of biological differences, especially sex-linked biology such as genital secretions, secondary sex characteristics and reproductive events like pregnancy or menopause. A wide range of genetic, hormonal and metabolic influences may play a part in shaping distinctive male and female patterns of morbidity and mortality. There is growing evidence of sex differences in the incidence, symptoms and prognosis of many health problems (Doyal 2001).

However, although biological factors such as genetics, prenatal hormone exposure and natural hormone exposure in adults may contribute to differences in men's and women's health, research combining both social and medical perspectives has concluded that a wide range of social processes can also create, maintain or exacerbate underlying biological health differences. Social and biological causes of differences in the health of women and men can 'amplify' or 'suppress' each other. For example, women have a stronger immune system and more flexible circulatory system to facilitate development of the foetus but, despite this biological advantage, they have lower life expectancy in many countries due to multiple social and economic disadvantages.

We may conclude that gender appears to affect the risks of mortality and morbidity through different exposure and vulnerability, the severity and consequence of illness, access to health promotion and the prevention, diagnosis and treatment of illness, health related behaviours, experience and implications of ill health, and finally the responses and accountability of the health sector. Gender equity in health must stand for the absence of bias that operates at many levels (Doyal 2001) within households (unequal recognition/treatment, economic differences in property, divisions of labour), community norms regarding women's and men's sexuality, reproduction and rights, and health providers, systems, policies and research.

Bias in gender and health research

There is a predisposition to focus research on the gender and health issues of developing countries, where the gender differences are extremely pronounced and the health delivery systems are largely inadequate in addressing women's health needs. For example, half a million women die every year as a result of pregnancy and virtually all these avoidable deaths occur in poor countries: this leads to the conclusion that women's reproductive health status is profoundly affected by who they are and where they live (Doyal 2000). However, the socioeconomic disparities in health even within developed countries are undeniable. The 1973-1993 period saw striking growth in income and wealth inequality in the USA and other developed nations, including an increase in the number of families living in poverty.

Socioeconomic inequality has been the mainstay of research around health inequity for more than a century. Socioeconomic factors, including education, income, income inequality and occupation have been identified as some of the strongest and most consistent predictors of health and mortality, and have been seen as more powerful than either sex or gender in determining health status. Nonetheless, although class may be an overall determinant of health inequalities, significant differences in health outcomes by race and gender remain within each level. Among the poor, female headed households are at a greater economic disadvantage because of the lower earnings of women and the dual nature of their work burden. This burden imposes severe time constraints, restricting such households' access to social and health services (Rosenhouse 1989). Within male headed households, the intrahousehold allocation of resources may have a gender bias, restricting women's access to adequate nutrition and health services. Power relations around sex and reproduction, and the complex intersections of class and gender, profoundly affect women's health seeking behaviour and health outcomes.

If health research does not explore the range of potential underlying factors that may contribute to social inequalities in health, the perception is reinforced that current ill health is inherent in the individual or social group. Consequently, policy solutions are formulated implying that the best intervention has to be at the individual level (such as addressing health behaviours and access to care) rather than transforming health delivery systems in order to improve the health of the population (Bird and Rieker 1999).

Gender and health research often focuses on intra-family role divisions and decision making processes. Since gender differences are more clearly observable in role divisions within the private sphere, health providers and policy makers often declare that gender inequalities are beyond their control and that they can only be addressed by profound societal change (Vlassoff and Moreno 2002). However, the power relations underlying gender differences are supported by diverse social institutions. It is therefore imperative that gender and health research examines the structural factors that contextualize individual agency within the larger political, social and economic framework.

There is still a lack of broad based multidisciplinary research that can examine both structural factors that affect inequitable health outcomes as well as gender power relations that directly influence health decision making and behaviour. Resources are needed to conduct more comprehensive research that can take historical, geographical, legal and political frameworks into account.

Some basic gaps in research on gender and health remain despite increased sophistication of methods. Firstly, data managers/systems are not doing even basic disaggregation by sex, let alone presentation of data to enable cross-tabulation between class, race, caste, ethnicity and other social differentials. Secondly, there is a serious lack of multidisciplinary research which can move out of the exclusive biomedical framework and study the social construction of health and well being as well as the socio-political determinants of ill health.

While clinical research is crucial to establish adverse impact of gender on women's health, it has been difficult to get recognition from health professionals of health problems that affect large numbers of women, for example reproductive tract infections or violence against women. This bias has led to research that dismisses women's complaints about pain and discomfort as either exaggeration and therefore unimportant, or as the norm, and therefore as 'medically insignificant' data. The collection of reliable data is also doubtful: health statistics based on official data from hospitals or health centres may underestimate women's mortality or morbidity because women often do not reach health centres for detection and treatment of their health problems. This often leads to the assumption that they suffer less from certain diseases when this is not the case (Vlassoff and Moreno 2002). Where gender bias exists in health seeking or where silent suffering is the norm, morbidity data will continue to be underestimated.

The concepts of gender and gender analysis which evolved from feminist research have not been mainstreamed into the training of health professional and researchers who are not exposed to these concepts and their importance to public health (Vlassoff and Moreno 2002). There is also a dearth of gender-sensitive research methodologies that can explore the qualitative dimensions of women's health as felt experience, rather than as an assumed biomedical construct. We have to start with the assumptions that gender differences in economic access, social power and behavioural norms operate, unless proven otherwise. The pathways can be complex and interactive but they can be investigated systematically.

Selected issues in gender and health

Gender and tropical medicine and epidemiology

Tropical medicine has often been characterized by its vertical nature. In the last decade, some epidemiologists have taken up the challenge to critically rethink the ways women, gender and oppression, and health are linked and studied. It is often assumed that the effects of tropical diseases on women and men are similar, with the proviso that women will suffer more acutely during pregnancy and childbearing (Rathgeber and Vlassoff 1993). The shortcomings of tropical medicine's approach to women and gender are the result of the fact that social scientists in tropical medicine also follow biomedical paradigms.

A gender framework for tropical diseases' research exists. In this framework, the variables of economic and productive activities, social-cultural activities and personal factors interplay with prevention, disease and the nature of treatment (Rathgeber and Vlassoff 1993). The question of why particular diseases affect particular individuals and groups is still not being fully addressed, leaving socio-cultural and political-economic analyses at the fringe. New methodological approaches have to illustrate how gender oppression shapes women's health and well being (Inhorn and Whittle 2001). If the problem definition and production of knowledge remain biased within mainstream epidemiological studies, women will continue to be biologically 'essentialized' as reproducers while women's health risks will remain decontextualized and depolitized (Inhorn and Whittle 2001).

Gender, power and inequality are strongly interrelated with the spread of infectious diseases. In 'Pathologies of power' (2005), Paul Farmer stresses that gender is one of the explanations of why so many women die of AIDS. Besides global ideologies that view women as inferior to men, poverty is a potential determinant in women's lives, causing suffering and inequalities (Farmer 2005). Other authors also challenge

contemporary epidemiological and biomedical research from a feminist and gender perspective. There are several examples of gender analysis of specific diseases, showing how stigma is experienced differently by men and women. This has implications for formulating interventions (Vlassoff and Moreno 2002). Integrating gender at the centre of health programmes requires:
- Creating awareness and understanding;
- Linking the social and biomedical sciences;
- Recognizing that gender inequalities are everyone's concern;
- Recognizing that medicine and health systems are gendered institutions;
- Linking gender to training and performance of health providers;
- Translating political will into resources for change; and
- Development and use of practical tools (Vlassoff and Moreno 2002).

In this sourcebook, research findings from Malawi are presented by Bertha Simwaka Nhlema and colleagues. Their study explores how gender roles and relations affect how key diseases of poverty are experienced at the community level. The question remains whether these studies and approaches have had any effect on the interventions targeting these diseases. Research and interventions addressing gender differences and inequalities are most common in the field of HIV/AIDS.

Gender and HIV/AIDS

Of the estimated 42 million people living with HIV/AIDS, women now constitute more than half of this number (Grown et al 2005). Given the particular vulnerability of women, the risk of women contracting HIV is rising worldwide. More than four-fifths of all infected women get the virus from their male sexual partner, often from their one partner (their husband). The remainder becomes infected by blood transfusions or from injecting drugs with a contaminated needle (Wegelin-Schuringa 2005). Women have a biological vulnerability but socio-cultural vulnerability contributes to the fact that women have a higher risk of being infected.

The culture of silence surrounding sex in many cultures, dictating that so-called good women are expected to be ignorant about sex and passive in sexual interactions, makes it difficult to inform women about risk reduction and negotiating safer sex (Gupta 2000). Gender norms also determine what women and men are supposed to know about sex and sexuality, and hence limit their ability to accurately determine their level of risk and to acquire accurate information and means to protect themselves from HIV.

In many societies, it is inappropriate for women to seek out or have extensive knowledge about sexuality or reproductive health. In addition, traditional norms of virginity for unmarried girls mean that they are poorly informed and puts them at a higher risk of being sexually abused. The emphasis on virginity of girls causes some of them to practise alternative sexual behaviour, such as anal sex, which also places them at a higher risk. Women's economic dependency also increases their vulnerability to HIV as it may lead to transactional sex for money or goods (Gupta 2000). This imbalance in power between men and women curtails women's sexual autonomy and expands men's sexual freedom, thereby increasing women's and men's risk and vulnerability to HIV (Gupta 2000).

Men are expected to be well informed about matters related to sex, although many are not. Norms with respect to masculinity can make it especially difficult for men to admit to this lack of knowledge. This applies even more to men having sex with men as this is deemed unacceptable in many cultures. This makes it difficult to seek and obtain information and services related to sexual health and protective measures (Wegelin-Schuringa 2005).

In the plenary address by Geeta Rao Gupta to the Thirteenth International AIDS Conference in 2000 in Durban, South Africa, the components of sexuality were described as the Ps of sexuality namely practices, partners, pleasure/pressure/pain and procreation and, last but not least, power. Practices refer to aspects of behaviour: how one has sex and with whom; the others refer to underlying motives. The power underlying any sexual interaction, heterosexual or homosexual, determines how the other Ps of sexuality are expressed and experienced. Power determines whose pleasure is given priority and when, how, and with whom sex takes place (Weiss and Gupta 1998; Gupta 2000).

Initially, only specific groups such as sex workers, intravenous drug users and homosexual men were considered to be at risk and the source of the spread of the HIV/AIDS epidemic. But, in time, the relationship between poverty and gender discrimination was known to represent major risk factors for HIV infection of women (Inhorn and Whittle 2001). At present, women, youth and men having sex with men are all considered to be at risk of becoming infected. In almost all societies, however, it continues to be impossible for women to negotiate for safer sex because of economic dependency and power relations.

This being the case, the worldwide-adopted prevention call of ABC (abstinence, being faithful and condom use) can be questioned. Without the power and skills to negotiate, women will not be able to protect themselves. In the 'State of the Population' report (UNFPA 2005), it is noted that ABC programmes do indeed expand awareness but only if women and men can make free and informed choices. ABC messages often overlook critical factors that millions of women are confronted with such as difference in age, respect, rape etc. The report asks: 'Does counselling abstinence until marriage keep young people safe when most are sexually active before they turn 20?' Indeed, it is clear that the so-called ABC (or AB) programmes have not led to an actual reduction in teenage pregnancies and HIV infections. One of the many alternatives to the ABC programmes is the RAP-rule of the Youth Incentives Project: a rights-based approach, acceptance of young people's sexuality, and participation of young people. In this sourcebook, Mabel Bianco and Miriam Zoll present innovative approaches with respect to HIV/AIDS.

Stigma

Stigma is another important issue in the context of gender and HIV/AIDS. Parker and Aggleton (2003) have provided a framework in their work on stigma and discrimination, arguing that stigma and discrimination in relation to HIV/AIDS can only be understood in terms of power and domination. In places where HIV is associated with sex between men or with drug use, the nature of the illness is often denied or those infected are abandoned for fear of being associated with the disease. Where HIV is seen as a sign of sexual promiscuity, the stigma is much higher for women than for men; they are much more likely to be expelled from their homes and families (Wegelin-Schuringa 2005).

Stigma is not only discrimination expressed by individuals but it is also a social phenomenon which builds on and strengthens existing differences. It is also used by dominant groups to legitimize and perpetuate inequalities such as those based on gender, age, sexual orientation, class, race or ethnicity. In this volume, Fiona Samuels and colleagues show how highly stigmatized groups in Indian society, such as female sex workers and men who have sex with men, can best be targeted through interventions.

Communities

Across the world, HIV positive women are more stigmatized and discriminated against than HIV positive men. Therefore, they underline a new emphasis on community mobilization and the need for structural interventions aimed at developing rights-based approaches to reduce HIV and AIDS-related stigma and discrimination (Parker and Aggleton 2003). In this volume, Madeleen Wegelin-Schuringa's article reflects on local responses to HIV/AIDS, presenting a toolkit which facilitates community mobilization.

What we can learn from HIV/AIDS is that the involvement of the community is crucial for successful interventions. In drought-stricken Swaziland, women who were active in food distribution were trained to address issues affecting the community such as sexual abuse, exploitation, AIDS and family planning. Community Relief Committees, consisting of 80% women, started discussing these issues in community meetings, churches etc. As a result, reporting of sexual abuse to the police, as well as testing of HIV and providing treatment, have all increased (UNFPA 2005).

At present, when more people have access to antiretroviral treatment (ART) than ever before, the reproductive choice of HIV positive people has become an issue, and services with respect to prevention from mother to child transmission are expanding. It seems essential that planners continue to increase gender sensitivity by reaching communities, and especially women and children.

One of the results of the HIV/AIDS pandemic is a larger interest in sexuality and sexual health. Although services on sexual and reproductive health and HIV/AIDS are not integrated as yet, and often the former receive less attention, the global focus on sexuality is now a fact. As Arnfred states in her latest work: 'The time has come for rethinking sexualities in Africa' (2005).

gender and health: policy and practice

Gender and sexuality

In the era of HIV/AIDS, the importance of better understanding of sexuality to improve sexual health becomes increasingly critical, and reproductive health remains one of the best entry points to achieve this. However, expanding reproductive health services to better address sexuality and sexual health issues continues to be challenging in many countries. There is still very little evidence of effective training of various cadres of health staff in counselling on sexuality and on how to sustain good quality counselling in sexual and reproductive health services (WHO/KIT 2006). As a result, despite best intentions to expand reproductive health services to the broader sexual and reproductive health (SRH) concept as prescribed in the ICPD Programme of Action, many programmes continue to struggle with the concept of sexuality.

Researchers studying sexuality often use narrow definitions of sexual behaviour, focusing almost exclusively on risks of pregnancy and disease. The analytical framework for studying sexuality and reproductive health should involve four dimensions of sexuality, namely sexual partnerships, sexual acts, sexual meanings, and sexual drives and enjoyment (Dixon-Mueller 1993). Other frameworks for studying sexuality concentrate on pleasure and desire, female agency, and the construction of femininity and masculinity (Arnfred 2005). In order to improve the effectiveness of prevention programmes for adolescents dealing with HIV/AIDS and teenage pregnancies, it is important to focus on the adolescents' own understanding and experience of their sexual behaviour. Female adolescents' experiences of their own sexuality are shaped by a range of contexts from intimate relationships to gender, ethnicity and class (Lesh and Kruger 2005).

This view is confirmed by a recent action research and awareness project in Benin carried out with and by 30 young people from 10-19 years of age, selected by their own communities. The outcome showed that, in addition to many questions and uncertainties about HIV/AIDS, teenage pregnancies and coercive factors surrounding them were seen as the biggest problem to be addressed (Kamminga et al 2005; Grown 2005). In this context, it is important to mention the current idea of sexual rights' advocates that sexual pleasure is a human right for both men and women. Here, a gender-neutral construction seems to emphasize more men's belief that they have a right to use women for sexual pleasure which is a recognized, cross-cultural barrier to effective HIV prevention.

Violence against women is fundamental to the construction of masculinity and is manifested through rape, social coercion, sexual objectification and prostitution. By challenging the forms of sexuality and sexual pleasure that reinforce masculinity, sexual rights should be formulated in such a way that they are based on sexual equality (Oriel 2005).

Violence against women

When discussing various challenges within the field of gender and health, violence against women needs to be discussed because it is a major public health problem and human rights' violation throughout the world. It is violence directed against women or girls on the basis of their sex. It includes acts that inflict physical, mental or sexual harm and suffering, threats of such acts, coercion and other deprivations of liberty (WHO 2002; WHO/KIT 2006). Most forms of violence against women and girls are related to gender inequality and to the desire to control women's sexuality. Sexual violence includes rape and other forms of sexual abuse and coercion, and may be perpetrated by partners, strangers, acquaintances or family members (WHO 2002; WHO/KIT 2006). It is difficult to know precisely the extent of sexual violence, but available data suggest that:

- In some countries, nearly one in four women is sexually coerced by her partner;
- Both boys and girls may be exposed to sexual violence in childhood;
- In some countries, up to one-third of adolescent girls report forced sexual initiation; and
- Each year hundreds of thousands of women and girls are bought and sold into prostitution (WHO/KIT 2006).

Characterizing women as a single, universal 'risk group', defined by reproductive biology epidemiology, seems to ignore the ways in which social realities of gender manifest themselves in women's bodies. Finkler has called these 'life lesions' and there are many examples of how gender relations get into the bodies of women, for example underweight babies, thinness and eating disorders, hypertension caused by day-to-day experience with racism and sexism, and experiences with gender violence such as female genital mutilation (FGM), and sex-selective abortion (Finkler 1994). In addition, women and girls who experience abuse may suffer severe physical and mental consequences, in both the short and the long term. In addition to the common physical consequences, including external and internal injuries, a number of acute and chronic sexual and reproductive health problems are associated with sexual assault, such as sexually transmitted infections (STIs), HIV, pelvic inflammatory disease, infertility, unwanted pregnancy, and sexual dysfunction (WHO/KIT 2006).

In this context, it also important to consider the practice of FGM, sometimes called female circumcision or female genital cutting, which comprises any procedure that involves the partial or total removal of the external female genitalia or other injury to the female organs for non-therapeutic or cultural reasons (WHO 1999). Worldwide, between 100 and 140 million women are currently affected. Every year, around 2 million girls and women are at risk of undergoing FGM. There are some reports that, where FGM was previously universally practised, the rates are now declining. However, among other groups, it has reportedly been introduced or revived (Shell-Duncan and Hernlund 2000; WHO/KIT 2006).

In the past, FGM was very much approached from a health perspective that was even used for convincing parents in Mali not to circumcise their daughters. Other discourses on FGM imply that the formation of gender identities, and the experience of pain as a marker of these identities, are contributing to the prevalence of the practice (Kwaak 2005). Globally, similar developments with respect to dealing with FGM seem to take place. Criminalization, harm reduction and opting for milder forms of FGM are visible processes worldwide. Moreover, there seems to be a gradual shift from emphasizing the medical complications to underlining girls' right to bodily integrity (Bocoum et al 2004). Most recently, it has been argued that interventions for preventing FGM from a public health perspective should be non-directive, culture-specific and multi-faceted if they are to be of any practical relevance (Jones, Ehiri and Ayanwu 2004).

The sexual and obstetric consequences of FGM have received most attention in the literature. A recent review of the evidence on the consequences of FGM for health and sexuality was based on sources published during 1997-2002 (Makhlouf Obermeyer 2005). It concluded that most studies appear to suffer from methodological shortcomings and that the available evidence does not support the hypothesis that FGM destroys sexual function or precludes enjoyment of sexual relations. There is evidence for increased risk of some complications of labour and delivery, as well as abdominal pain and discharge, but not for infertility and increased mortality of mother and child (Makhlouf Obermeyer 2005). What seems more relevant is that girls and women have the right not to be circumcised or harmed in any way.

The rights' perspective seems to be gaining more support. In a recent collection of articles by African authors, the Western approach to FGM is discussed (Nnaemeka 2005). Here, the authors claim their ownership of the practice and the problems related to it. In this sourcebook, Sehin Teferra presents successful strategies based on a rights' perspective and empowerment of women in the mitigation of FGM in Ethiopian communities.

Involvement of men

With respect to FGM, the argument for its perpetuation is often that it is a woman's issue in which men hardly have a voice. This does not seem to match reality because it is often men who need to marry a circumcised girl. Men, too, are fundamental in decision making processes at the household and community levels (Kwaak 1992, Bocoum et al 2004).

It is clear from the above discussion on the variety of topics in gender and health that the focus can no longer be on women only, women as a category without contextualization and diversification. In socio-behavioural studies in the field of HIV/AIDS, the emphasis on women only has found to be too narrow.

In 2001, Painter concluded that couple relationships have not been given adequate attention by socio-behavioural research in sub-Saharan Africa. For example, studies report that that voluntary counselling and testing (VCT) is associated with reduced risk behaviours and lower rates of seroconversion among HIV sero-discordant couples (Painter 2001). More and more authors are suggesting the need to reassess the pathways linking gender and health (McDonough and Walters 2001). In a review paper by the WHO, rates, barriers and outcomes are described for gender dimensions of HIV status disclosure to sexual partners. One of the outcomes is that efforts to promote couple counselling, thus involvement of the male partners, may help women to overcome barriers that they face to seeking VCT services (WHO 2004).

In addition to the assumed role of men in decision making processes with respect to health, or as the ones who are damaging the health of women through rape and sexual violence, there are other studies showing that men also have sexual and reproductive health-related information and service needs, similar to those of women. Both men's and women's needs may be best met through adherence to shared principles: focusing on educational, counselling and skills-building services, rather than on purely medical ones (Sonfield 2004). It is even observed that comprehensive reproductive health care seems to ignore one of its largest target groups, namely men.

Recently, more studies have been carried out with respect to the needs of men (Onyango-Ouma et al 2005; Parsons et al 2003). Within these types of studies, the construction of masculinity is an important issue, often discussed and linked to violence against women, sexuality and rape. Rape is presented as an act of punishment but also as an instrument of communication with oneself about masculinity and powerfulness (Jewkes et al 2005).

Gender analysis has been used to deconstruct notions of masculinity in South Africa. Such notions of masculinity are fluid, not limited to one category of men, and are also constantly defended and protected. In reality, as one speaks about multiple gender identities or femininities, one should also speak about masculinities, some of which support violent and oppressive gender relations, others which accept such gender relations, and still others which oppose them (Morrell 2001). A recent study from Southern Africa shows how men, in contrast to general perceptions, are positively involved in the care of HIV/AIDS patients and children, and financially support immediate and extended family members. They are at home, thereby enabling women to work and support other HIV or TB infected households (Montgomery et al 2006).

Another determining factor with respect to the successful involvement of men is that men might feel left out and even attacked by certain interventions. In this respect, work on the female condom as a marker of female empowerment is of interest. Women can use the female condom secretly and this is seen as a marker of the decrease of power of men and of empowerment of women. This issue needs to be addressed, in addition to financial barriers, if there is to be greater use of the female condom in Africa and elsewhere (Kaler 2001).

Within gender and health, it is clear that constructions of femininity and masculinity, and their various roles, responsibilities and power relations, need to be taken into account. Whether or not they are formulated in the Millennium Development Goals (MDGs), they are crosscutting realities from which one cannot escape. They determine the many gaps and challenges discussed in this introduction.

Gender and health in current international policy

From the 1980s onwards, a shift in policy approaches took place from Women in Development to Gender and Development. This shift acknowledged that gender analysis is key in the understanding of health, health seeking behaviour, health status, health planning and programming. Moreover, it was increasingly recognized that women and other vulnerable groups, lacking both a voice and equitable access to health care, should be involved at all policy and project levels. As a result of this, a so-called gender perspective became more widely known within development cooperation and within research, policy and practice, aiming at poverty reduction and a better health for all.

Since the ICPD in Cairo in 1994 and the UN World Conference on Women in Beijing in 1995, changing understandings of gender relations have evolved through research, brought to policy attention through advocacy and integrated in UN Declarations. Women's roles as producers, as well as visible and invisible forms of unpaid labour, are now recognized as having consequences for women's mental and physical health and well being. The sexuality of adolescents, knowledge of sexual and reproductive health, men's responsibility, gender-based violence and trafficking of women have been identified as having important implications for comprehensive reproductive health care, as does the rights-based approach.

Since the 1990s, gender mainstreaming has been seen as a strategy to find support for gender-sensitive interventions. In 2000, 189 countries met at the UN Millennium Summit to make a global pact against poverty. This pact led to the creation of the MDGs which were designed to be achieved in 2015. Goal 3 aims to promote gender equality and to empower women. Goal 4 aims to reduce child mortality and Goal 5 to improve maternal health. Reproductive health is directly related to these three MDGs but is not defined as an indicator of their success. Since Cairo, initiatives have taken place to reaffirm the ICPD Programme of Action. It is therefore remarkable to see that the agenda and outcomes of the Cairo Conference have not been translated into a separate MDG (Barton 2005; UNFPA 2005).

Some commentators state that many macroeconomic factors are undermining the Cairo Programme of Action. They link this to an increasingly conservative international environment and the predominance of World Bank policies. There seems to be an inherent contradiction between the goals of rights and equity in the health sector, on the one hand, and efficiency and cost effectiveness on the other (Ravindran and de Pinho 2005). Others have concluded that sexual and reproductive health and rights are not seen as determinants of gender equality in the context of the MDGs which focus, instead, on education for girls and maternal health and morbidity. This places women's and children's rights within a purely biological framework, addressing them as a vertical programme (Global Health Watch 2005).

Thus despite the changes outlined above, a gender approach is still not standard in the area of health and has still not been sufficiently integrated into the training of health planners and providers.

Conclusions

To conclude, applying the principles of gender equity in health policy and service delivery would first require understanding of different health impacts between women and men in terms of increased risks to ill health and decreased access to protective resources for health. One dimension in which this occurs is differential access to rights and resources, another is differential exposure to direct expressions of power such as violence, and a third is institutionalized disregard for women's biological needs and historical disadvantage. Gender equitable health policies would have to be primarily based on a commitment to protect and promote rights to health for all, acknowledgement of gender bias and the need to counteract it, accompanied by recognition of gender differentiated needs and associated constraints and barriers (Sen et al 2002). The significant differences in the health needs of women and men need to be clearly identified so that they can be reflected in equitable strategies for resource allocation.

The current climate focuses on shifting preventive health and care-giving responsibilities from state services to households. The current trend of health policies being framed by financial institutions has the inherent danger of making health into a technological and financially viable set of prescriptions that have little or no relevance to the vast majority of women. The dominance of bureaucrats, health technocrats and donor consultants has to be replaced by needs and rights based planning articulated by users and primary stakeholders. It is imperative to legitimize women's role in identifying and articulating their own needs, in planning, monitoring and evaluating health service provision.

The first conclusion drawn is that differences in health status for men and women are not merely biological but fundamentally affected by the social, political and economic forces that shape their lives, including unequal gender relations. Gender appears to severely affect:
- The risks of mortality and morbidity through different exposure and vulnerability;
- The severity and consequence of illness;
- Access to health promotion and the prevention, diagnosis and treatment of illness;
- Health related behaviours;
- Experience and implications of ill health; and
- Responses and accountability of the health sector.

Socioeconomic factors, including education, income, income inequality and occupation have been identified as some of the strongest and most consistent predictors of health and mortality. Gender inequity, combined with socioeconomic inequality, together form a powerful explanatory framework for variations in women and men's health. This implies that to understand health related differences between women and men, an analysis has to move beyond the health sector to look at the complex ways in which biology and social factors interact since social determinants exacerbate biological vulnerabilities.

Secondly, it is concluded that ill health is not inherent to the individual or social group but to the broader relations of power that provide the foundations of discrimination. Consequently policy solutions should rather focus on the more systemic transformation of larger social institutions to improve more equitable health outcomes and not remain at the individual level (addressing health behaviours and access to care). Individual agency needs to be contextualized within the larger political, social and economic framework.

In current health policy related approaches, it can be concluded that:
- The focus on institutional and financial reforms do not consider the gender implications of institutional reforms and neglect qualitative indicators to assess the gender impact;
- There is no recognition of women's unpaid work in the health care economy;
- Key beneficiaries and civil society organizations are still largely left out of priority setting and implementation;
- Increased community participation is more concerned with state withdrawal from direct service provision and health funding deficits than with empowering approaches that increase citizen voice along with provider accountability; and
- Gender inequalities in voice, power and influence continue to be neglected in the policy process (issues such as domestic violence, etc).

Applying the principles of gender equity in health policy and service delivery requires understanding of different health impacts between women and men in terms of increased risks to ill health and decreased access to protective resources for health, including differential access to rights and resources; differential exposure to direct expressions of power such as violence; and institutionalized disregard for women's biological needs and historical disadvantage. Gender equitable health policies would have to be based on:
- Commitment to protect and promote rights to health for all;
- Acknowledgement of gender bias and the need to counteract it;
- Recognition of gender differentiated needs and associated constraints and barriers; and
- Strategies that ensure equitable resource allocation.

Engendering health policy involves moving beyond equitable opportunities within the sector: it requires democratizing policy *processes* to the extent that users and their advocates are sufficiently informed and empowered to articulate their needs, claim these rights and pressurize systems to ensure gender-responsive outcomes. Experiences indicate that the engagement of a vibrant civil society constituency can exercise political pressure around the issue of gender equitable approaches in public policy.

This sourcebook

In the context of the previous discussion on gender and health, this sourcebook presents ideas, research and experiences from the wide field of gender and health in order to counteract some simplistic representations of this field. The articles here focus on topics that cannot directly be captured in the framework of the MDGs but which are of the utmost importance in the field of gender and health.

In the first article, Bertha Simwaka Nhlema and others synthesize the findings of a research programme in Malawi to explore how gender roles and relations affect how key diseases of poverty are experienced at the community level. The article documents strategies for translating gendered research findings into policy and practice. The authors conclude that it is clear that for both women and men, gender and poverty affect vulnerability to communicable disease, access to preventive and curative care, and the impact of disease at both an individual and household level. Greater cognisance of this at policy and practice level is vital in promoting gender equity in health.

Sehin Teferra presents various successful strategies in the mitigation of FGM in Ethiopian communities. She shows how the current role of women as the supporters of a practice that is designed to control and harm them, has to be replaced with a more positive role as empowered members of society. Any measures adopted either by the government, indigenous NGOs or community-based organizations must espouse the empowerment and rights of women as an overarching strategy in order to bring about sustainable change in the struggle against FGM.

Mabel Bianco describes how to reach teenagers through health messages and reproductive and sexual rights in Argentina. March 2003 saw the launch of a national Programme for Sexual and Reproductive Health throughout the country and, as a result of this, a study was carried out on communication. The study assessed sexual and reproductive messages targeted at adolescent populations in order to gain better knowledge and understanding of their rights to these services and to promote an enjoyable and safer sexual life. This article reflects on the findings of this study.

In the fourth article, Miriam Zoll underlines how complex and entrenched male-female gender systems are at the heart of the global HIV/AIDS pandemic. With more than 20 million deaths and 45 million infections, it is urgent that co-educational initiatives, involving both boys and girls, men and women, be incorporated into HIV prevention programming to challenge the established gender order and honestly explore heterosexual power dynamics. She sees opportunities for educating men and boys, and women and girls about the nuances of gender and sexuality, and for transforming this understanding into life-saving HIV prevention interventions. Such initiatives should include opportunities for groups of women and men to meet in single-sex as well as co-educational groups. She introduces the TRIZ approach and shows its merit from case studies in South Africa and Brazil.

In the fifth article, Madeleen Wegelin-Schuringa gives an analysis of programmes for local responses to HIV/AIDS that are documented in a toolkit which was developed by the Royal Tropical Institute in Amsterdam for UNAIDS (2004). She describes the gender implications of the lessons that can be learned from this analysis. The aspects covered are prevention through peer education; home-based care; involvement of people living with HIV and AIDS; the role of faith-based organizations; and approaches to increase sharing of knowledge and learning within countries.

Fiona Samuels and colleagues describe the nature, antecedents and the extent of stigma and discrimination among female sex workers and a cultural category of men who have sex with men in Andhra Pradesh, India. They have presented the findings of these two populations together because both involve strong gender dimension of stigma and discrimination. As is shown by this study and similar studies elsewhere, stigmatizing attitudes are the reflections of deep rooted and hierarchical social structures. Almost all the female sex worker respondents and most of the male respondents came from a poor socioeconomic background: relatively few were literate, and few reported having had the opportunity to develop any kind of life skills. Although the stigmatizing effects of poverty were reported by both groups of respondents, the burden was seen disproportionately higher in the female sex workers.

Acknowledgements

The authors would like to acknowledge with thanks the helpful comments of Madeleen Wegelin-Schuringa, MinkeValk and Maitrayee Mukhopadhyay on a previous draft.

References

Arnfred, Signe (ed.), 'Re-thinking sexualities in Africa'. 2nd ed. Uppsala, Almqvist & Wicksell Tryckeri, 2005.

Barton, Carol, 'Women debate the MDGs'. *Development* vol. 48, no. 1 (2005), p. 101-106.

Bird C.E. and P.P. Rieker, 'Gender matters: an integrated model for understanding men's and women's health'. *Social Science and Medicine* vol. 48, no. 6 (1999), p. 745-755.

Bocoum, Madina, Leon Bijlmakers, Dandara Kanté et Anke van der Kwaak, 'Étude sur les mutilations génitales féminines'. Plan Mali, 2004.

Boston Women's Health Book Collective, The new our bodies ourselves, (1992:14)

Correa, S., *Population and reproductive rights: feminist perspectives from the South*. London, Zed Books, 1994.

Cottingham, J. and C. Myntti, 'Reproductive health: conceptual mapping and evidence'. In: G. Sen, A. George and P. Östlin (eds), *Engendering international health: the challenge of equity*. Cambridge, MA, MIT Press, 2002.

Dixon-Mueller, Ruth, 'The sexuality connection in reproductive health'. *Studies in Family Planning* vol. 24, no. 5 (1993), p. 269-282.

Doyal, Lesley, 'Gender equity in health: debates and dilemmas'. *Social Science and Medicine* vol. 51 (2000), p. 931-939.

Doyal, Lesley, 'Sex, gender and health: the need for a new approach'. *British Medical Journal* vol. 323 (2001), p. 1061-1063.

Farmer, Paul, *Pathologies of power: health, human rights, and the new war on the poor*. Berkeley, CA, University of California Press, 2005.

Farr, William, First annual report to the Registrar General. London, Her Majesty's Statistical Office, 1839.

Finkler, Kaja, *Women in pain: gender and morbidity in Mexico*. Philadelphia, University of Pennsylvania Press, 1994.

Global Health Watch, 'B4: sexual and reproductive health'. In: Global Health Watch 2005-2006 report: an alternative world health report. London, Zed Books, 2005.
http://www.ghwatch.org/2005_report_contents.php

Grown, Caren, Geeta Rao Gupta and Rohini Pande, 'Taking action to improve women's health through gender equality and women's empowerment'. *Lancet* vol. 265, February 5 (2005), p. 541-543.

Gupta, Geeta Rao, 'Gender, sexuality and HIV/AIDS: the what, the why and the how'. Plenary address XIII International AIDS Conference, Durban, South Africa, July 12, 2000.
http://www.icrw.org/docs/Durban_HIVAIDS_speech700.pdf

Inhorn, Marcia C. and K. Lisa Whittle, 'Feminism meets the "new" epidemiologies: toward an appraisal of anitifeminist biases in epidemiological research on women's health. *Social Science and Medicine* vol. 53, no. 5 (2001), p. 501-567.

Jewkes, Rachel, Loveday Penn-Kekana, and Hetty Rose-Junius, "If they rape me, I can't blame them": reflections on gender in the context of child rape in South Africa and Namibia'. *Social Science and Medicine* 61 (2005), p. 1809-1820.

Jones, Susan D., John Ehiri, and Ebere Ayanwu, 'Female genital mutilation in developing countries: an agenda for public health response'. *European Journal of Obstetrics, Gynecology and Reproductive Biology* vol. 116, no. 2 (2004), p. 144-151.

Kaler, Amy, "It's some kind of women's empowerment': the ambiguity of the female condom as a marker of female empowerment'. *Social Science and Medicine* vol. 52 (2001), p. 783-796.

Kamminga, E., Edouard Wallace and Anke van der Kwaak, 'Summary of an adolescent sexual and reproductive health program formulation process with young people in the driver's seat (Couffo District Benin)'. Amsterdam/Cotonou, KIT, 2005.

Krieger, Nancy, 'Gender, sexes, and health: what are the connections: and why does it matter?'. *International Journal of Epidemiology* vol. 32, (2003), p. 652-657, provides twelve useful case studies to demonstrate the spectrum of situations where gender relations and sex-linked biology could affect exposure and health outcomes for women and men.

Kwaak, Anke, van der, 'Female circumcision and gender alliance: a questionable Alliance'. *Social Science and Medicine* vol. 35, no. 6 (1992), p. 777-787.

Kwaak, Anke, van der, 'Suffering, memory and globalisation'. Paper present at the ASA Conference, Washington, November 17, 2005.

Lesch, Elmien and Lou-Marie Kruger, 'Mothers, daughters and sexual agency in one low-income South African community'. *Social Science and Medicine* vol. 61 (2005), p. 1072-1082.

Macintyre, S., K. Hunt and H. Sweeting, 'Gender differences in health: are things really as simple as they seem?'. *Social Science and Medicine* vol. 42, no. 4 (1996), p.617-624.

Makhlouf Obermeyer, Carla, 'The consequences of female circumcision for health and sexuality: an update on the evidence'. *Culture, Health & Sexuality* vol. 7, no. 5 (2005), p. 443-461.

McDonough, Peggy and Vivienne Walters, 'Gender differences in health: reassessing patterns and explanations'. *Social Science and Medicine* vol. 52, (2001), p. 547-559.

Montgomery, Catherine M., Victoria Hosegood, Joanna Busza, and Ian M. Timaeus, 'Men's involvement in the South African family: engendering change in the AIDS era'. *Social Science and Medicine* vol. 63, (2006) (in press).

Morrell, Robert (ed.), *Changing men in Southern Africa*. London, Zed Books, 2001.

Mundigo, A.I., 'Men's roles, sexuality and reproductive health'. International Lecture Series on Population Issues. Chicago, Ill., The MacArthur Foundation, 1995.

Nnaemeka, Obioma (ed.), *Female circumcision and the politics of knowledge: African women in imperialist discourses*. London, Praeger, 2005.

Oriel, Jennifer, 'Sexual pleasure as a human right: harmful or helpful to women in the context of HIV/AIDS'. *Women's Studies International Forum* vol. 28 (2005), p. 392-404.

Onyango-Ouma, W., Harriet Birungi, and Scott Geibel, 'Understanding the HIV/STI risks of men having sex with men in Nairobi, Kenya'. Horizons, Frontiers in Reproductive Health. Nairobi, Population Council, 2005.

Painter, Thomas M., 'Voluntary counselling and testing for couples: a high leverage intervention for HIV/AIDS prevention in sub-Saharan Africa'. *Social Science and Medicine* vol. 53 (2001), p. 1397-1411.

Parker, Richard and Peter Aggleton, 'HIV and AIDS-related stigma and discrimination: a conceptual framework and implications for action'. *Social Science and Medicine* vol. 57 (2003), p. 13-24.

Parsons, J.T., P.N. Halkitis, R.J. Wolitski, C.A. Gomez, and the Seropositive Urban Men's Study (SUMS) Team, 'Correlates of sexual risk behaviours among HIV-positive men who have sex with men'. *AIDS Education and Prevention* vol. 15, no. 5 (2003), p. 383-400.

Rathgeber, E. and C. Vlassoff, 'Gender and tropical diseases: a new research focus'. *Social Science and Medicine* vol. 37, no. 4 (1993), p. 513-520.

Ravindran, T.K. Sundari and Helen de Pinho (eds.), 'The Right reforms? Health sector reforms and sexual and reporductive health'. Johannesburg, Womens' Health Project, School of Public Health, University of Witwatersrand, South Africa, 2005.

Rosenhouse, Sandra, ' Identifying the poor: is 'headship' a useful concept?'. *Living Standards Measurement Study Working Paper no. 58*. World Bank, Washington, D.C., 1989.

Sen, G., A. George and P. Östlin (eds), *Engendering international health: the challenge of equity*. Cambridge, MA, MIT Press, 2002.

Shell-Duncan, B. and Y. Hernlund (eds), *Female 'circumcision' in Africa: culture, change and controversy*. Boulder, CO, Lynn Rienner, 2000.

Sonfield, A., 'Meeting the sexual and reproductive health needs of men worldwide'. *The Guttmacher Report on Public Policy* vol. 7, no. 1 (2004), p. 9-12.

UNFPA, 'State of world population 2005. The promise of equality: gender equity, reproductive health & the MDGs'. New York, NY, United Nations Population Fund (UNFPA), 2005.

Vlassoff, C. and C. García Moreno, 'Placing gender at the centre of health programming: challenges and limitations'. *Social Science and Medicine* vol. 54 (2002), p. 1713-1723.

Wegelin-Schuringa, Madeleen, 'Factsheet: Gender and HIV/AIDS'. In: Resource pack on gender and HIV/AIDS. Geneva/Amsterdam, UNAIDS/KIT 2005.

Weiss, E. and G. Rao Gupta, 'Bridging the gap: addressing gender and sexuality in HIV prevention'. Washington, DC, International Centre for Research on Women (ICRW), 1998.

WHO, 'Female genital mutilation: information kit'. Geneva, World Health Organisation (WHO), 1999.

WHO, 'World report on violence and health.' Geneva, World Health Organization (WHO), 2000.

WHO, 'Gender dimensions of HIV status disclosure to sexual partners: rates, barriers and outcomes'. Geneva, World Health Organization (WHO), 2004.

WHO/KIT, 'Integrating sexual health interventions into reproductive health services: programme experience from developing countries'. Geneva and Amsterdam, World Health Organization (WHO) and Royal Tropical Institute (KIT), 2006.

introduction

Bertha Simwaka Nhlema, Ireen Makwiza, Lifah Sanudi, Patnice Nkhonjera and Sally Theobald

1 Engendering communicable disease policy and practice: experiences from Malawi

This paper synthesizes the findings of research in Malawi to explore how gender roles and relations affect the way in which key diseases of poverty are experienced at the community level. The paper also documents strategies for translating gendered research findings into policy and practice. First, it highlights background information on Malawi and gives an overview of the three key diseases of poverty. Next, it introduces the Research on Equity and Community Health (REACH) Trust and documents its research work on gender and equity in diseases of poverty. This is followed by a conceptual framework on how gender shapes vulnerability to diseases; access and adherence to services; and the impact of being ill on individuals and households. Strategies for facilitating the uptake of gender-sensitive research findings in the design of policy and interventions are then analysed.

Diseases of poverty in Malawi

Malawi has a population of about 10 million people (National Statistical Office 2000). It is one of the poorest countries, rating 157th out of 174 countries on the Human Development Index of the United Nations Development Programme (UNDP). According to the latest Malawi Poverty Profile, 65% of the population is poor (National Economic Council 2000). Malawi's poor are not a homogeneous group but consist of a cross-section of the population including smallholder farmers with less than one hectare of land, estate tenants, urban poor and female-headed households. Their principal coping mechanism is *ganyu* labour, a range of short-term rural labour relationships. About 40% of households are headed by women, and most of these households are poor.

Malawi's mortality pattern is typical of a developing country. It has very poor health indicators with a high proportion of deaths caused by infectious diseases like tuberculosis (TB), malaria and the human immune deficiency virus/acquired immune deficiency syndrome (HIV/AIDS) (Government of Malawi 2004). Malaria is the leading cause of outpatient visits (30%) and is a leading cause of under five mortality (40% of deaths) (Government of Malawi 2001b). The number of TB cases has risen from 5,334 in 1985 to 22,674 in 1998 (WHO 1999), reflecting a rise from 82 per 100,000 per annum to 193 per 100,000 per annum. The increase in the TB incidence has partly been attributed to HIV/AIDS.

HIV/AIDS constitutes a serious threat to the country as a whole as it has affected all the aspects of Malawi's social and economic fabric. There are approximately one million people infected with HIV in Malawi (Government of Malawi 2004). AIDS causes approximately 81,000 child and adult deaths annually and is the leading cause of death in the reproductive age group (20-49 years).

The Ministry of Health is the main health service provider in Malawi, accounting for 60% of health services, followed by the Christian Health Association of Malawi (CHAM) with 25% (Government of Malawi 2001b). The remaining 15% of services are provided by private for profit and non-profit organizations. In the government facilities, most services are free of charge at the point of delivery.

Introducing the REACH Trust

The Malawian National TB Programme (NTP) has an excellent record and international reputation for conducting programme-relevant operational research. In 1999, the NTP formed a research collaboration with the Liverpool School of Tropical Medicine, UK, and the University of Malawi to expand the operational research base. This research collaboration was funded by the British Department for International Development (DFID) as the TB Equity Project, with the aim of conducting research to promote access to TB care, particularly for the poorest and most vulnerable. The project was based on the principles of interdisciplinary research, research capacity building and ongoing dialogue with policy and decision makers. Under the TB Equity Project, a number of research studies on gender, poverty and TB and on barriers to access to TB care were conducted. Since 1999, the collaboration has expanded into a programme of research to promote equity in TB, attracting additional core funding from DFID in addition to project grants from TDR Project, Stop TB Partnership, the Norwegian Heart and Lung Association and EQUINET, Southern Africa.

In 2004, the programme submitted its registration as an independent Malawi research trust called REACH. Part of the Trust remains the Equi-TB Knowledge Programme, a research collaboration which provides technical support to the Trust from the Liverpool School of Tropical Medicine. The Trust aims to promote strategies that enhance the delivery of health services for the poor, vulnerable and disadvantaged, through the conduct of research in the major diseases of poverty including TB and HIV/AIDS, and to promote equity in the provision of care and treatment for these diseases.

Methods

Thew REACH Trust has conducted research on access to health care services using multiple methods. It has applied complementary qualitative and quantitative methods to document context specific barriers to accessing health care services from community, patient and health worker perspectives. Specific methods employed included focus group discussion with community members and TB, HIV/AIDS and malaria patients. Individual in-depth interviews were also conducted with TB and HIV/AIDS patients, key informants and other stakeholders. Follow-ups of patients who had defaulted from treatment were undertaken as well. Structured interviews using a questionnaire were conducted with TB patients to quantify costs and delay in seeking care. Gender analysis was carried out in all studies to allow in-depth analysis of the impact of power and social relations on access to services and adherence to drug regimens. A synthesis of the findings from these studies is presented in the section 'How gender roles affect key diseases at the community level'.

Linking with policy makers and practitioners

The results from these studies were used to recommend potential interventions for ensuring poverty and gender-sensitive approaches in disease control. Consultations with stakeholders, including policy makers and providers, informed the creation of the research agenda, research methods and strategies for disseminating findings. Stakeholders included the NTP, the National AIDS Control Programme, the HIV/AIDS Unit within the Ministry of Health, the National Malaria Control Programme, district health offices, the city assembly and The Lighthouse – a charitable trust implementing the Government of Malawi supported antiretroviral therapy (ART) programme. The ways in which the REACH Trust has tried to ensure the research findings are fed into policy and practice are documented in the section 'Translating gendered research into policy and practice: challenges and opportunities'.

How gender roles affect key diseases at the community level

Gender analysis provides a useful tool for critically examining and unpacking power relationships in society, and adds an important dimension in poverty and vulnerability analysis. Gender refers to men and women's characteristics, which are socially and culturally determined (Williams et al 1994; WHO 1998). It is related to how men and women perceive themselves and each other, and how we are expected to think and act as men and women because of the way in which society is organized.

This section will document the relationship between gender roles and relations and the key diseases of poverty in Malawi (TB, HIV/AIDS and malaria) at the household and community level. The way in which gender roles and relationships shape the following will be discussed: vulnerability to disease; access and adherence to services; and impact of ill health on individuals and communities. These linkages are illustrated in Figure 1.

Gendered vulnerability to TB, HIV and malaria

Traditionally ill health has been, and continues to be, associated with poverty and vulnerability. Poverty and vulnerability are multifaceted and shaped by gender roles and relations which impact on power, voice and participation in social structures (Narayan et al 2000). Biological factors, gender divisions of labour and the gendered nature of poverty lead to differential risk and vulnerability to HIV, TB and malaria for women and men (Bates et al 2004).

Gendered disparities in HIV infection are particularly stark in the younger age groups. For example, younger women are more vulnerable to acquiring HIV infection than men, partly for physiological reasons such as immature genital tract and high rates of asymptomatic untreated STIs in young women. In sub-Saharan Africa, there are on average 13 infected women for every 10 infected men (UNAIDS 2004). The prevalence of HIV/AIDS amongst young women aged 15-24 is four to six times higher

Figure 1: Conceptual framework

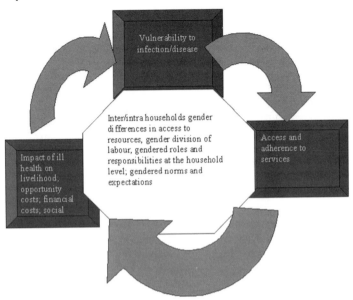

Vulnerability to infection/disease

Inter/intra households gender differences in access to resources, gender division of labour, gendered roles and responsibilities at the household level; gendered norms and expectations

Access and adherence to services

Impact of ill health on livelihood; opportunity costs; financial costs; social

than amongst young men of the same age (National AIDS Commission 1999). These differences have been attributed to the way in which gender shapes an individual's ability to negotiate safe sex against a backdrop of poverty and violence.

With regard to gender differences in TB incidence, globally there are 1.7 times as many male pulmonary TB cases reported annually as female cases (WHO 2001). Some evidence suggests that this may be due to gendered inequities in access to care, with women facing a number of barriers in accessing TB services (Hudelson 1996). The male: female TB ratio in Malawi is similar to the global notification rates trend, and is 1.08:1 (WHO 1999). However, the trend varies from district to district, with some districts presenting high notification rates for women and others low.

Malaria is a major cause of illness amongst the general population in Malawi, with an estimated 40% of the admissions and 30% of all hospital deaths in under-five children being due to malaria and associated complications (Government of Malawi 2002). Women with lower levels of education are more likely to have fever than women with higher levels of education (National Statistical Office 2000). Malaria is frequently referred to as a disease of the poor or a disease of poverty. Gwatkin and Guillot (2000) demonstrated that 58% of the malaria deaths occurred in the poorest 20% of the world's population, a higher percentage than for any other disease of major public health importance.

Access and adherence to services: a gender analysis

Accessing care presents challenges for poor men and women. Gender roles and relations result in differential access to resources at household and community level. The ability to make decisions over resources for accessing care is vital. It has been documented that in most developing countries men decide on the allocation of resources for the care of a family member in times of ill health (Taylor et al 1996).

Analysis of pathways to seeking care in Malawi reveals that women take longer to report to health facilities than men. The delay period amongst TB patients showed that women took longer to be diagnosed with TB than men, and had more repeated visits to health facilities. The barriers to seeking care are more complicated for poor women, possibly due to lack of power in decision making over resources. Before visiting public facilities, patients shop around between different care providers, such as storekeepers, private providers and public health facilities for treatment. The trend is similar for HIV/AIDS and malaria. Qualitative assessments of pathways for care seeking for malaria revealed that storekeepers are the first contact providers for treatment, although in most cases women need to seek permission to use resources for buying drugs for fever from men. In addition, repeat visit to health facilities due to the long diagnosis process and also lack of proper diagnosis lead to huge costs to patients.

Financial and opportunity costs of accessing care have been identified to be major barriers to early diagnosis and treatment of TB and HIV/AIDS. The costs of accessing care are increased due to system related barriers such as the need for repeat visit to the health facility for diagnosis and treatment, and lack of speedy laboratory diagnosis techniques.

In addition, access to resources at household level also affect adherence to treatment and may lead to dropping out of treatment and diagnosis. In-depth interviews with patients on TB treatment and ART showed that patients usually have to bear transport costs for both themselves and their guardian, namely friends or relatives who escort the patient whenever they go to the health facility. Financial constraints were also cited as the main barrier to adherence to treatment. There was some evidence from qualitative research at The Lighthouse that where men are the breadwinners, they are likely to prioritize access to ART drugs for themselves, while women faced financial barriers in accessing care. In a context of limited resources and costly drugs, individuals and families have to make very difficult decisions about who should have access to ART.

In addition, social stigma associated with illness such as HIV/AIDS and TB sometimes acts as a barrier to seeking care and adhering to services. HIV/AIDS is stigmatized because of the strong relationship to sex, and by implication loose sexual behaviour, and TB because of its perceived relationship with HIV/AIDS. The fear of stigma can prevent patients who have symptoms suggestive of HIV/AIDS and TB from seeking care. Qualitative studies conducted suggest that women suffer more social consequences from HIV/AIDS and TB than men. Disclosure of a positive HIV status has led to some women being divorced by their husband and social isolation.

Impact of ill health on individuals and households

Measures put in place to cope with the cost of accessing care push households into greater poverty, especially those that are poor and are female headed. For example, information from individual in-depth interviews with TB patients revealed that poor men and women sell their assets and take heavy interest loans known as *katapila* to cope with the burden of ill health. There were notable gender differences between female headed households and male headed households, the problems being worse within the former. Besides selling assets, most of the female headed households in urban settings had to stop buying water from communal taps and resorted to using water from traditional wells. This exposes them to other illnesses, such as diarrhoea and skin diseases. As one female respondent notes:

> Since the illness we stopped buying a whole bag of maize per month, instead we buy a pail of maize. It is now several months since we stopped using the communal public water tap because we couldn't pay, we now use water from the traditional well after illness.

In Malawi, patients' families and households are directly affected in two ways when seeking health care. Firstly, someone has to act as their guardian at the clinic or hospital and, secondly, someone has to replace their activities in the home. The patient himself or herself has to forgo his or her livelihood activity. As in most countries, the role of caring in Malawi is mainly done by women. Women have to make the decision to either escort the patient to the hospital/health centre, or continue with their livelihood activities. It is clear that a patient's female relatives spend significantly more time acting as guardians for TB patients (7 working days per month) than their male relatives (4.3 days per month). In total, female family members are used as guardians 60% of the time, compared to male family members (37% of the time). Women are thus more likely to lose income-earning opportunities than men.

While patients are seeking health care, often someone else in the household has to fulfil their everyday tasks. This person is frequently their spouse, potentially resulting in further income loss, or a child, resulting in lost education. Men were less likely to have their activities replaced than women (70% of men had no one replacing them, compared with only 30% of women). The poor were more likely to have no one replacing their activities than the non-poor.

Most of the parents who did not have older female relatives, their domestic activities were replaced by children, and mostly by female children. Women's activities, in particular, were replaced by children. Many of those children who replaced the role of their mother had to miss attending school.

Gendered roles, relations and differential access to resources at household level not only lead to vulnerability to infections or diseases but also to ability to access and adhere to drug regimens. The impact of health seeking and ill health is also impoverishing; poor women and men may become extra vulnerable to ill health due to reduced access to clean water and food. Hence there is need to employ gender and poverty approaches across the whole spectrum of health responses: from prevention to cure.

Summary of how gender shapes vulnerability, access and impact of ill health
- Gender roles and access to resources shape both the ability of men and women to access care and the impact of ill health. In Malawi women have less power to make decisions on resources for accessing services. This is a similar trend to other developing countries. In the qualitative assessments it was found that women have to seek their husband's approval or at least notify them before incurring any expense.
- Also affected by TB and HIV/AIDS are guardians who provide caring activities to patients.
  · Most of these guardians are women: it is a common trend in Malawi for men to leave caring activities to women.
  · Studies also revealed more financial costs for female guardians because they had to travel with patients more than male guardians.
- Opportunity costs were higher for women and girls who had to take up caring roles than men. Some of the girls had to drop out of school to concentrate on caring for their mums.

Translating gendered research into policy and practice: challenges and opportunities

There are substantial obstacles to translating research findings into policy and practice (United States Department of Health and Human Services 2002). The relationship between policy and practice is not linear or straightforward (Groenewald 2005); we cannot assume that more research means more evidence based policy. We have identified a complex myriad of opportunities and challenges in translating gendered research into policy and practice. Key to this are four inter-related themes that are explored in turn (1) working in a participatory way with policy makers, practitioners and community members; (2) advocating research findings at strategic forums; (3) multi-method approaches; and (4) 'strategic framing' – adopting different languages or discourses to discuss gendered research findings.

Working in a participatory way with policy makers, practitioners and community members

As discussed in the section 'Introducing the REACH Trust', the REACH Trust has grown out of a research relationship with the NTP and other partners. Its relationship with the NTP is further strengthened as the head of NTP is the Reach Trust director; it shares premises and sits on all NTP strategic management groups. This means that Reach Trust and NTP have been able to work together in identifying research gaps, designing and implementing research projects, and discussing the implications of research for policy and practice. This strong relationship is illustrated through the following two case studies.

Davis and Howden-Chapman (1996) argue that research findings are more likely to be translated into policy and practice if 'researchers involve managers and policy makers in the development of the framework for and focus of research and if investigators assume a responsibility for seeing their research translated into policy'. The case studies have shown how working closely with the NTP has created an opportunity for translating research findings into interventions that meet the gendered needs of poor women and men, as well as developing strategies to institutionalize, and hopefully sustain, a gendered approach in NTP's core business.

Case study 1: Translating gendered community needs into practice: working with storekeepers

The findings from poor women and men's pathways to seeking care for TB were fed back to community members using participatory approaches, including drama. In the ensuing discussion, community members proposed a community-based intervention to shorten the pathway and hence enhance their access to TB services. They suggested that storekeepers and key community members should be equipped with advisory and health promotion skills since they are first contacts in care seeking, being easily accessible at the community level. The proposal was then presented to providers and policy makers at district and national level through different forums such as conferences and management meetings for the NTP. The community members proposed that addressing barriers should not be limited to TB, but that malaria should also be included because it is a major health problem for children, women and men. Mothers and female carers in particular face challenges and opportunity costs in seeking care for children with symptoms possibly indicative of malaria, as caring is constructed as a largely female role. Consequently discussions were also held between the National Malaria Control Programme and the NTP. A joint malaria-TB intervention was developed to address issues of improper advice on home management of malaria and delay in seeking care for TB. The intervention involves training storekeepers, volunteers and community members in health promotion and referral skills, and early evaluations show that women's participation is higher compared to men. The majority of volunteers are women and women form 50% of all health committees.

Case study 2: Integrating gender equity and concerns into NTP core business

Through advocacy from the REACH Trust, the NTP has also strengthened its institutional capacity through creating a post in Gender and Equity. The post holder is expected to sustain collaboration, analysis and dissemination of gender disaggregated data for advocacy. The programme integrated equity and gender within their five years development plan from 2001 to 2006. This included, for example, setting aside funding for community-based initiatives to address barriers and costs of accessing care. With the current focus on decentralization in the Malawian health sector, the NTP is using the findings of these community-based initiatives to advocate that districts need to incorporate community-based activities within their District Implementation Plans.

Advocating research findings at strategic forums

Our work on barriers to access and adherence to ART was conducted at the time of policy discussions on how to scale up ART across Malawi. We presented our findings showing that cost constituted the key barrier to access to ART and that this was gendered, with women in particular struggling to meet the costs required, at a number of key policy discussions groups and strategic fora. Through participation at a number of strategic working groups, our findings fed into discussion at the Ministry of Health and were arguably influential in shaping the Malawian policy (drugs provided free on a first come first served basis, with a particular emphasis on health promotion strategies that are geared towards poor and vulnerable groups).

Multi-method approaches

Health research that contributes to change may require more methodological pluralism (Davis and Howden-Chapman 1996). REACH has used multiple methods including quantitative approaches (questionnaires, gender analysis of pre-existing routinely collected health information) and qualitative approaches (focus group discussions, in-depth critical incidence interviews and participant observation). The REACH Trust has found that presenting findings from multiple methods can be strategic in advocating change. This comes down to both personal preference (some policy makers prefer and are more convinced by quantitative methods and vice versa) but also opportunities to present a holistic picture. For example, analysis of questionnaires can produce statistical significance on the numbers of poor women and men failing to access services; whilst the qualitative findings can help explain and contextualize these figures by describing in poor women's own words the barriers, challenges and obstacles they face in service access. Qualitative testimonies can be a powerful tool in highlighting gendered disparities in health experiences.

Strategic framing: adopting different languages or discourses to discuss gendered research findings

We have found that it can be strategic to situate research findings within different languages or discourses depending on the audience. This has been referred to as 'strategic framing' and has been discussed in the gender literature (see Theobald, Tolhurst, Elsey, Standing 2005; Theobald, Tolhurst and Squire 2005; Pollack and Hafner-Burton 2000). As individuals we may believe and work within a gender equity and rights discourse, i.e. poor women have a right to accessible and quality TB services, but we may choose to situate our research findings within instrumental or technical arguments that prioritize *efficiency or sustainability*, as these may be more accessible to policy makers than a discussion of gender and rights. It could, for example, be argued that if TB services are inaccessible or unacceptable to poor women, TB programmes will be unable to meet their case finding and cure rate targets, with negative repercussions for the community of a large number of untreated, infectious TB cases: this clearly threatens the *efficiency and sustainability* of the entire TB programme.

Concluding comments

Gender-sensitive research approaches help to highlight inequities in access to resources to promote and protect health (Baume et al 2001) with implications for health sector responses. The research findings clearly illustrate how gender roles and relations affect not only vulnerability to TB, HIV and malaria, but also access and adherence to services and the impact of disease on individuals and households in Malawi. The multiple ways in which gender and poverty intertwine to shape health experiences and outcomes need to be realized and acted upon if health policy and practice is to be equitable, efficient and sustainable. This is not a straightforward process and research findings are not a passport to policy (Davis and Chapman 1996).

For research findings to inform policy and practice, there is a need for well thought through strategies and approaches. Key to this is the importance of developing sustained and responsive relationships with policy makers. This enhances the ownership of the research process and hence the likelihood of policy makers adapting policy and practice in the light of research findings. Other strategies to promote uptake of gendered research findings include sustained advocacy at policy fora and technical working groups that uses multiple methods (numbers and voices) to illustrate the main issues and deploy different strategic frames – equity, gendered rights, efficiency, sustainability – depending on the audience. Whichever arguments we find most compelling, it is clear that for women and men, gender and poverty affect vulnerability to communicable disease, access to preventive and curative care and the impact of disease at both an individual and household level. Greater cognisance of this at policy and practice level is vital in promoting gender equity in health.

References

Baume, E., J. Mercedes, and S. Hillary, 'Gender and health equity resource guide'. Brighton, Gender and Health Equity Network, 2001.
http://www.ids.ac.uk/ghen/resources/papers/Geneq.pdf

Bates, I., C. Fenton, J. Gruber, D. Lallo, A.M. Lara, S. Bertel Squire, S. Theobald, R. Thomson, and R. Tolhurst, 'Vulnerability to malaria, tuberculosis, and HIV/AIDS infection and disease. Part 1: determinants operating at individual and household level'. *The Lancet Infectious Diseases* vol. 4 (2004), p. 267-277.

Davis, P. and P. Howden-Chapman, 'Translating research findings into health policy'. *Social Science and Medicine* vol. 43, no. 5 (1996), p. 865-872.

Groenewald, C., 'Translating research into policy'. 2005. Downloaded from
http://population.pwv.gov.za/ConSemEvents/Documents/TranslatingResearchIntoPolicy%20-%20Cornie%20Groenewald.doc (accessed October 2005)

Government of Malawi (GoM), 'Malaria policy'. Lilongwe, Ministry of Health and Population, 2002.

Government of Malawi (GoM), 'Malawi roll back malaria: five years strategic plan, 2001-2005'. Lilongwe, Ministry of Health and Population, 2001a.

Government of Malawi (GoM), 'National health accounts'. Lilongwe, Ministry of Health, 2001b.

Government of Malawi (GoM), 'The programme of work, sector wide approach'. Lilongwe, Ministry of Health, 2004.

Gwatkin, D.R. and M. Guillot, 'The burden of disease among the global poor: current situation, future trends, and implications for strategy'. Washington, DC, World Bank, 2000.

Hudelson, P., 'Gender differentials in tuberculosis: the role of socio-economic and cultural factors'. *International Journal of Tuberculosis and Lung Disease* vol. 77 (1996), p. 391-400.

Narayan, D., R. Patel, K. Schafft, A. Rademacher, and S. Koch-Schulte, *Voices of the poor: can anyone hear us?* Washington, DC, Oxford University Press for the World Bank, 2000.

National Economic Council, 'Profile of poverty in Malawi 1998: an analysis of the Malawi Integrated Household Survey, 1997-1998'. Zomba, National Statistical Office, 2000.

National Statistical Office and ORC Macro, 'Malawi demographic and health survey 2000'. Zomba, and Calverton, Maryland, National Statistical Office and ORC Macro, 2001.

National AIDS Commission, 'Malawi national HIV/AIDS estimates'.1999.

Pollack, M. and E. Hafner-Burton, 'Mainstreaming gender in the European Union'. *Journal of European Public Policy* vol. 7, no. 1 (2000), p. 432-456.

Rajeswari, R., R. Balasubramanian, M. Muniyandi, S. Geetharamani, X. Thresa, and P. Venkatesan, 'Socio-economic impact of tuberculosis on patients and family in India'. *International Journal of Tuberculosis and Lung Disease* vol. 3, no. 10 (1999), p. 869-877.

Taylor, L., J. Seeley, and E. Kajura, 'Informal care for illness in rural south west Uganda: the central role that women play'. *Health Transition Review* vol. 6, no. 1 (1996), p. 49-56.

Theobald, S., R. Tolhurst, and S.B. Squire, 'Gender, equity: new approaches for effective management of communicable disease'. *Transactions of the Royal Society of Tropical Medicine and Hygiene* vol. 100, no. 4 (2006), p. 299-304.

Theobald, S., R. Tolhurst, H. Elsey, and H. Standing, 'Engendering the bureaucracy? Challenges and opportunities for mainstreaming gender in Ministries of Health under sector-wide approaches'. *Health Policy and Planning* vol. 20, no. 3 (2005), p. 141-149.

UNAIDS, '2004 Report on the global AIDS epidemic'. Geneva, UNAIDS (Joint United Nations Programme on HIV/AIDS), 2004.

United States Department of Health and Human Services, 'Translating research into practice (TRIP)-II. Fact sheet'. *AHRQ Publication* no. 01-P017. Rockville, MD, Agency for Healthcare Research and Quality, 2001. http://www.ahrq.gov/research/trip2fac.htm (accessed October 2005)

WHO, 'Gender and health: a technical paper'. *WHO/FRH/WHD/98.16.* Geneva, World Health Organization (WHO), 1998.

WHO, 'Global tuberculosis control'. *WHO/CDS/TB/2001.287.* Geneva, World Health Organization (WHO), 2001.

WHO, 'Putting research into policy and practice: the experience of the Malawi National Tuberculosis Programme'. *WHO/CDS/CPC/TB/99.268.* Geneva, World Health Organization (WHO), 1999.

Williams S., J. Seed, and A. Mwau, *The Oxfam gender training manual.* Oxford, Oxfam, 1994.

2   Tackling tradition: examining successful strategies in the mitigation of female genital mutilation in Ethiopian communities

How can I refuse to get my daughter circumcised when no one will marry her if she is not 'pure'? Who will make sure she will eat?
(A project participant in 2003)

A *seratuma* is a traditional form of meeting by which the Oromo people of Ethiopia determine major decisions affecting the community. In these meetings, the elders of the clan pronounce joint decisions that are often questioned and debated by all present until a general consensus is reached. During one *seratuma* in Arsi Negelle in April 2001, clan elders asked a group of girls who had come to attend the meeting if they thought the practice of female genital mutilation (FGM) that had been practised in the community for generations should be continued. When the question was met with a resounding 'no' from the girls, the elders declared the practice unlawful for any community member henceforth.

On this occasion, the elders called for this particular *seratuma* following a series of workshops on gender relations facilitated by Hundee, an indigenous NGO working in Oromia, the largest region in Ethiopia. In these workshops, the workload, access and control of resources by men and women are analyzed, with a special emphasis on traditional practices that harm women, such as abduction and FGM. A strategy that Hundee has found to work very well has been to involve youth as well as parents and teachers in the fight against FGM. In Arsi Negelle Zone where women are traditionally circumcised just before marriage, Hundee has found that girls who have been empowered to speak out against the practice after attending its workshops are refusing to be circumcised. The impact of this development in terms of challenging both the practice and women's status in the community has been great.

This paper examines some of the successful strategies used by indigenous Ethiopian NGOs such as Hundee in eradicating FGM. The central focus of this study is the identification of best practices that can be replicated by other organizations working in similar fields in Ethiopia and elsewhere as appropriate. The paper also investigates the impact of the work of these NGOs on gender relations in the communities in which they operate with the hope that some indigenous NGOs and funding agencies may find the compilation of a number of successful strategies of use.

The field research for this paper took the form of case studies examining the work of three indigenous NGOs working in different parts of Ethiopia to mitigate FGM, focusing on their successful strategies and investigating the impact of their work in reducing gender inequality in their respective areas.

Conceptual framework

The use of the term 'female genital mutilation' in this paper is intentional. Following the argument posed by the Foundation for Women's Health Research and Development (FORWARD) that 'any definitive and irremediable removal of a healthy organ is mutilation' (Shell-Duncan and Hernlund 2000), the term emphasizes the political nature of the practice and shows that FGM is a deliberate and violent procedure that is designed to control women's sexuality and, by extension, women themselves. The term calls attention to the harmful impact of the practice on the lives of women and illustrates the fact that FGM is one of the extreme ways in which some societies control women and girls. Although the word 'mutilation' might be taken to denote condemnation, its criticism is targeted not at communities or individuals, but rather at the patriarchal manifestation of institutions such as the family and marriage that justify the practice and encourage women to be its most ardent supporters.

What is FGM?

The term FGM refers to all procedures that involve partial or total removal of the external female genitalia for cultural, religious or other non-therapeutic reasons (WHO 2000). Although the exact origins of the practice are not known, references to FGM have been found in the ancient civilizations of Egypt and Sudan. There is some speculation that it originated at the time of the pharaohs as indicated by the term 'pharaonic circumcision'. The practice, which was maintained for thousands of years, was eventually incorporated into Islam and spread to other countries along with the religion, leading to the unfortunate assumption that it is a requirement for good Islamic practice (Gruenbaum 2001). However, FGM is not limited to Muslims; Christians, Animists and Ethiopian Jews also practise it.

Each year, two million girls are at risk of undergoing FGM. It is practised primarily in 28 African countries, in a small minority group in India, and also among some migrant populations in Western countries (Toubia 1995). Forms of FGM were also practised in the UK and the USA as recently as the 1950s to 'treat' 'hysteria, lesbianism, masturbation and other so-called female deviances' (Toubia 1995).

In general, the main reasons given by parents for having FGM performed on their daughters are to reduce sexual desire of women in order to ensure chastity, virginity and, ultimately, fidelity during marriage (Gruenbaum 2001). The sociological reasons for the practice include the initiation of girls into womanhood and the maintenance of social cohesion (Gruenbaum 2001). In many traditional societies as well as some immigrant communities in the West, virginity is often a prerequisite for marriage and thereby economic security and societal acceptance. In such communities where a woman's level of sexuality usually denotes her moral standing, FGM has become an essential component of womanhood.

Effects of FGM

In addition to the severe physical pain and trauma caused by the actual procedure, the immediate health consequences of FGM may include shock, haemorrhage, tetanus infection, urine retention, as well as acute and chronic urinary tract infection. In addition, possible complications often lead to genito-urinary problems such as difficulties with menstruation and urination, pelvic inflammation, painful menstruation, injury to adjacent organs, broken bones, ulceration and infections that sometimes result in death. Long-term consequences include infertility, dermoid cysts and abscesses, scar formation, painful sexual intercourse and difficulty during childbirth. For example, post-partum haemorrhage is shown to be significantly more common among women who have undergone FGM. The cause for the increased haemorrhage is the incisions made and the perineal tears experienced as a result of the scarring from FGM (WHO 2000). In addition, many women who have undergone FGM suffer from its psychological after-effects such as anxiety and depression (WHO 2000). The effects of FGM vary according to the type of procedure and the extent of the damage it causes.

FGM in Ethiopia

The National Committee on Traditional Practices in Ethiopia (NCTPE) carried out a national baseline survey in 1997/1998 with the objective of establishing an information base that would enable it to identify targets, draw up policies and develop strategies to combat harmful traditional practices (NCTPE 2003). The survey showed that 72.3% of the female population in Ethiopia has undergone some form of FGM. The prevalence found ranged from 94.5% in the Afar Region to 70.2% in the capital, Addis Ababa. The survey showed that FGM is practised in almost all parts of Ethiopia and is prevalent in 46 out of 82 ethnic groups. There is speculation that FGM, together with male circumcision, came to Ethiopia with the introduction of Judaic practices a few centuries before the birth of Christ. In Afar in particular, it is considered to have been introduced by the Ancient Egyptians with whom the Afar are known to have had contact (NCTPE 2003).

Cliterodectomy (Type I and the simplest form of FGM) is the most prevalent type of FGM accounting for 62% of all cases, followed in prevalence by excision, which is the removal of the clitoris together with partial or total removal of the labia minora (Type II). Infibulation (Type III), the removal of part or all of the external genitalia and stitching or narrowing of the vaginal opening allowing only for the flow of urine and menstrual blood, is practised on 3% of the female population (NCTPE 2003).

The type of procedure and the age at which it is done varies according to the region and ethnic group. In general, among populations that perform Type I and Type II, the procedure tends to be done as early as the eighth day after birth. This is also the case for Afar where infibulation is the most prevalent type of FGM. In other areas, including parts of Oromia, girls are circumcised between the ages of five to ten. Some ethnic groups such as the Kembatta have girls circumcised as adolescents, usually just before marriage (NCTPE 2003).

In most cases, an older woman who also acts as a birth attendant performs the procedure. In parts of Oromia, where girls are circumcised between the ages of five and ten, the procedure is traditionally preceded by a feast prepared by the mother. Where FGM is performed on adolescents, for example in Kembatta and neighbouring

Sidama Zones, the girl sits on a stool with her head and arms held back while her bridesmaids cover her eyes with both hands. The circumciser, sitting or squatting, faces the girl with the cutting instrument. The process is more complicated in case of infibulation. After the clitoris and other parts of the genitalia are carved away by the circumciser, the sides of the labia majora are usually held together and a paste made up of traditional herbs is applied to the wound to promote healing. The thighs are then tied together and the girl is left lying on a mat until the wound has healed. By that time, the vagina opening will be closed except for a tiny opening left for passing urine. The vagina is usually not opened again until the girl gets married when her husband defibulates her using a sharp instrument (NCTPE 2003).

FGM is prevalent both among Orthodox Christian and Muslim Ethiopians, with a slightly higher rate among Muslims (NCTPE 2003). As in other parts of the world where it is practised, FGM is imbued with cultural significance and is associated with religious obligations, even though it is not prescribed by any religious texts. For instance, in some parts of Ethiopia, Orthodox priests have been known to refuse to baptize girls who have not undergone some form of FGM (personal communication from community members in Western Shoa Zone, Oromia, February 2004).

A survey done by NTCPE found that in Ethiopia, public awareness of the consequences of FGM is inversely proportional to the support of the practice. In general, awareness of the harm caused by FGM, and support for its eradication are higher in urban areas. In addition, resistance to the eradication of the practice tends to be stronger in areas of high prevalence levels (NCTPE 2003). Despite its pervasiveness and cultural significance, FGM in Ethiopia is being challenged from many sides with local and indigenous NGOs often at the helm of the struggle.

In search of strategies

The field research for this paper, undertaken over a two-month period in 2004, consisted of a combination of focus group discussions and semi-structured, in-depth interviews with community members and leaders, NGO representatives as well as traditional birth attendants and circumcisers.

The three NGOs profiled in this paper were chosen based on their impressive track records in tackling FGM in their respective areas, and because they are all indigenous organizations staffed by men and women from the same ethnic group as the communities, putting them in a unique position to question and challenge their own traditions. All three have been successful in channelling their ties to the communities they serve to foster faith in their work and, to varying degrees, have achieved a sense of community ownership of their programmes and projects.

Identifying similarities and differences between the three makes it possible to draw common themes and best practices on working against FGM. The most effective strategies identified by the three indigenous NGOs surveyed in this research (and corroborated by the research undertaken in their programme areas) are summarized below.

Kembatta Mentii Gezzima – Tope

Kembatta Mentii Gezzima – Tope (KMG) was founded in 1997 in Kembatta-Alaba-Tembaro Zone in the Southern Nations, Nationalities, Nations and People's Regional State of Ethiopia. Described as 'an indigenous, non-governmental, women-centred, integrated community development organization' (UNDP 2003), KMG works in the areas of reproductive health, HIV/AIDS, FGM, gender-based violence, civil and legal literacy as well as vocational training and livelihood programmes for women. KMG addresses FGM in the context of gender issues, women's health and human rights (KMG 2001).

KMG is perhaps best known for its work with young men and women who become role models for their peers by either refusing to undergo FGM, or getting married without the woman undergoing the procedure. In fact, the highly publicized wedding of a young woman from Kachebirra *Woreda* (district) who had refused to be circumcised showed the programme's involvement of the youth in the campaign against FGM. At the wedding, the bride wore a placard stating that she was happy to not have been circumcised and the groom wore one affirming that he was happy to marry an uncircumcised woman. Over 2000 people attended the wedding (KMG 2002).

Successful strategies used by KMG include:
- Promoting progressive interpretation/implementation of existing laws at all levels, combined with public education. The NGO emphasizes the legal aspect of traditional practices such as FGM, and has played a major role in persecuting a number of circumcisers and parents who have had their daughters circumcised in recent years. The activism shown by KMG in pushing for the imprisonment of FGM practitioners lends credence to the argument made by the Ethiopian Women Lawyers Association (EWLA) that progressive implementation of the existing laws could go a long way towards mitigating FGM (Ashenafi 2000).
- Encouraging young men and women to be role models who inspire collective action against FGM. The first couple that married without the woman having been circumcised has become a source of inspiration for thousands of their peers in Kembatta.
- Involving community stakeholder institutions, such as churches and schools, that can play important roles in giving legitimacy to the effort to end FGM. For instance, KMG organizes sensitization workshops for teachers that in turn educate their students about the harmful effects of FGM; and clergy in the area have been known to speak out about FGM and other harmful traditional practices.

Hundee

The indigenous NGO Hundee, which is operational in five zones of Oromia region, gets its name from the Oromiffa word for 'root' or 'base', denoting its grass-roots approach to development. Hundee was founded in 1995 with the purpose of serving marginal communities. The work of Hundee is based on respect for and revival of aspects of the Oromo culture, and aims to foster community ties at every level. Recently, the work of Hundee has extended to civic education centred on women's rights and harmful traditional practices. The latter consists of workshops on gender

tackling tradition

and leadership, as well as on harmful traditional practices such as rape and abduction.

Successful strategies used by Hundee include:
- Conducting participatory workshops where community members debate issues. Hundee has found that discussion forums where men and women community members (made up of community leaders as well as others with less influence on public opinion) are encouraged to bring up the complex issues that surround FGM, have led to community-owned decisions against FGM. This strategy is also applied by KMG.
- Supporting peer education by community members. Volunteer members of Hundee and KMG are doing wonderful work in sharing information with their neighbours, communities and *idirs*, namely traditional associations where a group of people contribute money into a common pool that is then given back to individual members to aid with the cost of weddings, funerals and other social events. This is also used by KMG.
- Facilitating the creation of a 'critical mass' of men and women who actively oppose FGM, and who act as self-appointed regulators to ensure that community decisions against FGM are adhered to by all. The NGO has found that empowered men and women are often willing to be on the forefront of the efforts to stop FGM.

Afar Pastoralist Development Association

Afar Pastoralist Development Association (APDA) is one of a few indigenous NGOs run by Afar nationals. It operates in four out of five zones of Afar, the least developed of all Ethiopian regions. APDA has a holistic view of development and has programmes in literacy, non-formal education in pastoral settings and primary health care, including the health needs of women. In addition, APDA conducts activities aimed at HIV/AIDS prevention and educates against traditional practices affecting women and children. APDA views FGM as one of the many traditional practices that harm women and promote inequality between men and women.

As the profiles indicate, all the NGOs view FGM as a manifestation of gender inequality in their respective communities. All three have gender components in their goals, although their approaches vary widely. For instance, while KMG (and to a lesser degree, Hundee) actively promote women's empowerment as one of the main tools for stopping the practice in addition to sensitizing the community at large and health providers, APDA does not use this approach at all. Instead, it advocates against FGM from the perspective of educating the community about the harmful effects of the practice on women's health.

Successful strategies used by APDA include:
- Using visual materials such as videos to emphasize the physical damage caused by FGM. This strategy has greatly aided the work of all the NGOs in creating visual imagery of FGM and has helped create important breakthroughs for APDA. This strategy has had a powerful impact on men in particular, as they are usually not aware of the extent of the damage done by the practice.

- Teaching that there is no religious basis for FGM. In Afar in particular, the most important reason given for FGM is the belief that it is a practice required by Islam. Refuting this notion has had a large impact on challenging FGM. Furthermore, training religious leaders to act as change agents has had significant impact where teachings by *qadis* (Islamic religious leaders) have been instrumental in helping the community challenge FGM.
- Connecting education about the harmful effects of FGM with its risk of transmitting HIV/AIDS. This strategy is especially effective in light of the national information campaign on HIV. This strategy is also used by Hundee.

Findings

The impact of the work of each NGO is visible to varying degrees. Kachebirra, the *Woreda* selected for this field study, has a highly successful anti-FGM programme funded by GTZ (German Agency for Technical Co-operation). In this district, there has been a real breakthrough in terms of mitigating FGM. The strategy of targeting adolescents to stand against FGM has borne significant fruit. Since KMG started its intervention in the area in 1999, 6865 women have pledged to not undergo FGM, and close to 50 women have married without being circumcised. The general consensus from the interviews and focus group discussions was that FGM is on a definite decline here.

Ejere *Woreda*, Western Shoa zone, is the location of one of Hundee's GTZ-funded programmes. According to the participants of the focus group discussion, FGM has been completely abandoned in the area since the *seratuma* or traditional meeting that was held on the subject in 2000. The community is now working to stop other harmful and patriarchal practices such as marriage by abduction. Marriage by abduction, a common practice in many parts of the country, happens when a man abducts and rapes a young woman (usually in her teens), forcing her to marry him as she is no longer considered eligible for marriage to another man. As with FGM, abduction is currently being challenged by NGOs and citizens' groups.

While the research did not include a formal quantification of the level of success achieved so far by the NGOs in question, there seemed to be the least change in Afar. For instance, one circumciser reported that although she no longer performs infibulations as she has learnt from APDA of the harm caused by the practice, the number of requests that she receives has not decreased significantly. The strategy adopted by APDA is different from the other two NGOs. Based on the reasoning that the community would reject any suggestion that it stops all forms of FGM at once, APDA recommends the substitution of infibulation with the milder *sunna* circumcision or excision (Type II FGM where the clitoris is completely removed together with the partial or total excision of the labia minora). The first focus group discussion showed a general consensus that through the seminars held by APDA, the community has a new awareness of both the harm caused by FGM and the fact that it is not a religious requirement. There is consensus that if infibulation is to be stopped, only excision *(sunna)* can replace it because, as one clan leader informed the researcher, failure to circumcise either girls or boys is considered *haram* (sinful) in the community's understanding of Koranic teaching.

However, *sunna* is considered to be acceptable from the perspective of both religious teaching and the girl's health. The impact of this change was seen in one participant's explanation that once she found out that infibulation was not a religious requirement, she decided to not have her two young daughters infibulated. Instead, she has had them left 'open' (unfibulated but excised).

Sustainability

Impact analysis in the three programme areas identified that the FGM programme in Kachebirra Zone has had the largest impact in changing people's attitudes. Turning to the issue of the sustainability of the changes made in the community, all the participants agreed that there is still much work to be done to maintain the momentum of change. One participant expressed concern that the information that KMG supplies has not reached everyone in the community, and that he hoped that KMG would continue to work hard to bring about sustainable change. All the participants agreed that the continued presence of KMG in the community was essential for ensuring that the flow of information about the harm caused by FGM.

Despite the sense of ownership of the activism against FGM and other harmful traditional practices by the community, none of the focus group participants thought that the schools, churches and legal institutions that are influential in the community could maintain the work by themselves.

In an effort at sustaining the community's decision to stop the practice of FGM, Hundee sets up 'women's rights' defence committees' in each sub-district made up of district officers, school teachers and directors, local women's affairs office staff as well as volunteers from the community. The committees are charged with following up on any violation of community decisions made to stop the practice. Also, the community-owned decision to give up the practice is made sustainable by workshop attendees who are undertaking peer education of their neighbours and members of their *idirs* and passing on information about the harmful effects of FGM.

Conclusions

This research provided a brief 'snapshot' of examples of how local and indigenous NGOs such as APDA, Hundee and KMG are working with the men and women of their communities to question and challenge harmful traditional practices such as FGM. It is important to link the above discussion of successful strategies in mitigating FGM with the initial presupposition that the work done by these NGOs would be incomplete without a fundamental challenge to the gender status quo. This paper asserts that the most important strategy for challenging harmful traditional practices such as FGM is allowing women the space and the opportunity to empower themselves and others in their communities. FGM is a patriarchal practice, based on the belief that a woman's sexuality, with its implication for the family's honour and the institution of marriage, needs to be controlled. It is therefore a practice that cannot be completely dismantled until women are empowered to realize their fundamental human and reproductive rights.

Women's complicity in FGM is a result of ingrained patriarchy that devalues women and their role in society. Entrenched patriarchal attitudes have convinced many Ethiopian women that their value rests in their relationships with men. As mothers, aunts and grandmothers who are concerned that their charges are 'pure' and marriageable, women are often the staunchest supporters of the continuation of the practice. The current role of Ethiopian women as the supporters of a practice that is designed to control and harm them has to be replaced with a more positive role as empowered members of society. Any measures adopted either by the government, indigenous NGOs or community-based organizations must espouse the empowerment of women as an overarching strategy in order to bring about sustainable change in the struggle against FGM.

References

Ashenafi, Meaza et al, 'Harmful traditional practices affecting the health and rights of women: law reform as strategy for change: a report'. Addis Ababa, National Committee on Traditional Practices of Ethiopia (NCTPE), 2000.

EWLA (Ethiopian Women Lawyers Association), 'Activity report November 1999-December 2000'. Addis Ababa, EWLA, 2001.

Gruenbaum, Ellen, The female circumcision controversy: an anthropological perspective. Philadelphia, PA, University of Pennsylvania Press, 2001.

KMG, 'Update Kembatta Women's Center/Ethiopia'. Addis Ababa, Kembatta Women's Self-Help Center (KMG), Vol. 2 (June 2001).

KMG, 'Update Kembatta Women's Center/Ethiopia'. Addis Ababa, Kembatta Women's Self-Help Center (KMG). Vol. 3 (October 2002).

NCTPE, 'Old beyond imaginings: harmful traditional practices in Ethiopia'. Addis Ababa, National Committee on Traditional Harmful Practices of Ethiopia (NCTPE), 2003.

Shell-Duncan, Bettina and Ylva Hernlund (eds), 'Female 'circumcision''. In: Africa: culture, controversy and change. London, Lynne Rienner Publishers, 2000.

Toubia, Nahid, 'Female genital mutilation: a call for global action'. New York, Research, Action and Information Network for Bodily Integrity of Women (RAINBO), 1995.

UNDP (United Nations Development Programme), 'Interview with Dr. Bogalech Gebre, Director of Kembatti Mentti Gezzima – Tope (KMG). Partnership to fight poverty'. UNDP Ethiopia Newsletter vol. 13, no. 3 (2003).

WHO, 'A systemic review of the health complications of female genital mutilation including sequelae in childbirth'. WHO/FCH/WMH/00.2. Geneva, World Health Organization (WHO), 2000.

3 Reaching young people on health and reproductive and sexual rights: the experience of Argentina[1]

Argentina is a country with a strong Catholic tradition although other churches and religions are recognized. From the early 1970s, family planning activities were forbidden, both in public health services and social security health services. This prohibition was restricted in 1986 by a National Government Decree but, with the change of Government, strong opposition developed once again from 1989 onwards so that such services were once again curtailed (Bianco 1996). In addition, no sex education was provided at school to teenage girls and boys. As a consequence, sex and sexual issues remained taboo in schools and often within families too. At the same time, these issues were liberally and openly presented in the mass media, especially on television and radio.

In December 2001, the political and social crisis led to the resignation of the National Government and three successive national governments in less than a month. Finally, a provisional government was designated by the parliament, remaining in power for two years until general elections were held. The year 2002 was characterized by an increase in poverty with the proportion of people living under the poverty line increasing from 20% to 60% (Bianco et al 2003). This was largely due to the economic crisis and resulting mass unemployment, brought about by the devaluation of the peso.

The crisis also led to the collapse of the public health services, the reappearance of malnutrition and an increase of other diseases. A significant rise in infant mortality, maternal mortality rates and adolescent pregnancy was also observed, with rape and sexual abuse becoming increasingly present in the news. These trends led to the re-opening of the discussion on the need for a national law on sexual and reproductive health in the Senate. The law was passed in the Representative Chamber in mid-2001 but was not accepted by the Senate until October 2002 when, due to the deterioration of sexual and reproductive health, the national Government and the Senators eventually decided to pass it. The law created the national Programme of Sexual and Reproductive Health within the Ministry of Health, and established services in all the provinces, including sex education in public schools. The law stipulated that adolescents should have access to public services, allowing the provision of contraceptives and other methods of contraception (http://www.conders.org.ar). Previous to this law, access to advice and provision of contraceptives was extremely difficult. Adolescents did not have access to the public health services and were not able to procure contraceptives through the national health system. As a result, only those with the means to pay for private services had access to contraception.

March 2003 saw the launch of a national Programme for Sexual and Reproductive Health throughout the country. Within this framework, *Fundacion para Estudio e Investigacion de la Mujer* (FEIM), in collaboration with the National Network of Adolescents and Young People for Sexual and Reproductive Health (REDNAC) carried out a study on how to communicate sexual and reproductive messages to young people, aged 15-24 years, in order for them to gain better knowledge and understanding of their rights to these services, and to promote an enjoyable and safer sexual life. This study provides the focus of this paper.

Characteristics of the study

The REDNAC network was created in 1999 and by 2004 had 23 member groups and organizations (http://www.rednacadol.org.ar). The study reported in this paper focused on four geographical areas, each one with different characteristics that are representative of different socio-cultural contexts. We chose two areas in the North of the country, one in the Northeast and the other in the Northwest, both with very conservative traditional societies, strongly influenced by the Catholic Church. The other two areas comprised Greater Buenos Aires, the capital of Argentina, which has the most open and liberal society; and the southern region, characterized by new population settlements from other parts of the country and from neighbouring countries. Settlers in the southern region have moved principally for economic reasons, and they are less dominated by tradition and more open to new ways of life.

In these four areas, we interviewed a reference population such as teachers, professors, health workers, journalists and government personnel, all working with young people. The interviews were carried out by members of the network, namely local young people from each area especially trained for this purpose. FEIM researchers designed a special questionnaire in order to collect information on this reference population's opinions on:
- the status of the sexual and reproductive health of young people;
- the needs of young people; and
- organizations in the region working in the field of sexual and reproductive health and rights.

As part of this study, news published in national and local newspapers on issues relating to sexuality and adolescents' sexual and reproductive rights and health was also studied.

Workshops for young people aged 15-24 years old were organized to discuss their own understanding of their status and needs related to sexuality, sexual and reproductive rights, and health. These workshops trained the participants in communication techniques and methods. They were asked to develop messages and communication material in order to promote sexual and reproductive health and rights among young people. The messages and communication products produced by the young people in the four areas were tested on groups of local young people. The resulting communication material was compared, focusing on how to effectively inform and promote a healthy and safer sex life for young people.

Sexual and reproductive health issues in the media

In three of the four geographical areas studied there was very little news in the media on sexual and reproductive health issues. Where such news was broadcast, it related principally to HIV/AIDS prevention but did not, for example, include the promotion of the use of condoms. In the two northern areas of Argentina, the few articles published in the last year were about HIV/AIDS prevention. In the Northwest, only one article about adolescent pregnancy was published, and the comments came from Catholic Church groups or conservative politicians. Furthermore, a discussion about the approval by law of the National Sexual and Reproductive Health Programme led to many articles in local newspapers opposing the approval of the national programme. However, this did not affect the implementation of the national programme in the state public health services.

In the southern area, the local newspaper included articles and information about HIV/AIDS prevention programmes developed by the state government, NGOs and local authorities. A few articles relating to adolescent pregnancies and sexuality were found, but these demonstrated much less bias than was found in the Northwest. In Greater Buenos Aires, many articles and reports in the three principal newspapers mentioned sexuality, sexual rights and health of young people, teenage pregnancies, male adolescents' sexual attitudes, habits and activities, as well as research and studies developed by governments, NGOs, universities, schools and young people. Many opinions and editorials were published, demonstrating a variety and diversity of perspectives.

In conclusion, we found the issue was not very often present in the state and local newspapers and, when present, was generally only linked to HIV/AIDS prevention. At the national level, the issue was fully covered by the principal newspapers, and expressed the interest of the population and the government. As a general rule, there is no presence of a special section in newspapers where young people can voice their opinions, so their opinions and comments are hard to find.

Adults speaking about young people on their behalf is the rule. This strongly exemplifies the tendency in Argentina not to consider young people as subjects of rights and for them to not be taken fully into account. They are still considered children and are therefore not allocated the space and rights to express themselves independently. They are, however, actually not treated as children, but are considered responsible for their acts including being penalized legally when committing mistakes, a serious contradiction with serious consequences.

A further point is that very little distinction is made between girls and boys in the media. The gender issue among young people is not highlighted or explored. Instead, the media strengthen existing prejudices by commonly using images and messages that portray young females as erotic subjects.

reaching young people on health and reproductive and sexual rights

57

Adults' perceptions of the status and needs of young people

As part of this study, a selection of 48 adults was interviewed. These adults considered that the sexual and reproductive health of young people was 'average' or 'poor' due to: lack of health services provided to young people; lack of sexual education in schools and other forms of information; and the high level of teenage pregnancies. Very few mentioned irresponsibility as a cause of these issues. Many mentioned the lack of policies focusing on either young people or sexual and reproductive health. Common health problems identified were teenage pregnancies, sexually transmitted diseases (STDs) and violence, including sexual violence.

When we explored what adults consider to be the best and most effective methods to communicate messages on sexual and reproductive health to young people, there is a general consensus that television and community activities are by far the most effective. The Internet was also mentioned but only as a secondary method. In terms of themes, teenage pregnancy and HIV/AIDS prevention came up as top priorities. The majority of these messages currently follow the line of normative messages, namely focusing on what young people should or should not do, rather than educating them to make informed decisions. A further aspect is that, in general, young women are the main target of the information diffused, with much less being aimed at young men, especially in the younger age bracket. As such, the sample of adults interviewed demonstrates the traditional gender perspective with girls seen as being responsible for reproductive health and contraception.

With respect to condom use, there is a tendency to direct messages to the male rather than female population. In general, adults do have the decision power as to whether or not to have sexual relations but the decision to use condoms or not is taken by men, while women decide on methods of contraception. This shows how gender roles in Argentina are perceived. There are currently no signs of concrete proposals to stimulate a discussion on these themes with parents, teachers and young people.

Young people's own ideas and proposals

In each area with REDNAC members' participation, a group of young people of both sexes, aged between 15-24 years old, were invited to participate in a workshop. This involved training on sexual and reproductive health, and rights and sexuality issues. Information about communication and mass media in general was included. The participants were asked to decide which issues they would prioritize, what messages they wanted to articulate and which form of communication they would use.

Some 75 young people took part in the workshops, 56% of whom were female and 44% male, with an average age of 18 years. Most of the participants were students in their last years of secondary school or first year of university or college. In Greater Buenos Aires, participants were younger than in the other three areas. The participants identified the following priorities: sexual and reproductive rights; use of contraceptives; myths about sexuality; and non-discrimination in relation to sexual preferences. These issues did not match those put forward by adults, nor with those presented in the newspapers. Identification of these issues did demonstrate their need for information as well as interest in the topic, and the fact that they were not adequately reached by their schools, media or the governmental programmes.

There were, however, some gender differences in the identification of priorities. Girls tended to give more importance to reproductive rights, rights to information access, as well as methods of contraception and clarifying its usage; while boys gave more importance to sexual rights, condom use and HIV/AIDS. Both groups emphasized non-discrimination in terms of sexual preference, HIV/AIDS infection, age, and socioeconomic status. Young people in Argentina are most sensitive to any form of discrimination and are themselves subject to discrimination at a time when social attitudes are suspicious of young people, especially young males. Young males are, by virtue of their sex and age, suspected of many kinds of transgression and inadequacy. This is also demonstrated by the actions of the police force and their manner of addressing young men.

Radio was identified as the preferred medium for receiving messages, particularly certain community radios rather than the more commercial ones. Radio allows more interaction, where young people can call in by telephone and participate in dialogues with the audience. It is important to emphasize that through radio, young people do have the opportunity to speak out and express opinions. This is something that never happens in newspapers or on television. On community radio, young people are considered to comprise actors and subjects, and their opinions and comments are welcomed. They did not therefore agree with adults that the best channel of information transmission is television. They also did not agree with the idea of community activities, nor with the use of leaflets as mentioned by adults as being of prime importance. All young people interviewed also clearly agreed that the Internet is a good method and a good second option in order to reach young people and transmit messages. They also consider the use of banners and posters in schools to be good, especially in sporting encounters and other places where young people meet.

Messages developed by young people

Each group came up with two or more messages. They were also assessed on how they communicated the final messages. FEIM provided technical assistance and financial support in order to supply the elements enabling the production of these messages. The issues tackled in these projects varied according to the area as well as the age and gender constitution of the groups.

In Greater Buenos Aires, sexual and reproductive rights were viewed as lacking because of problems in the access to health services, contraceptive methods and the way HIV/AIDS prevention was being handled. It should be noted also that the four groups in this area were younger than in the other regions; all were aged between 14-17 years old.

The adolescents produced posters to be displayed in schools with a box to allow people to ask questions they would then answer. Other posters referred to methods of prevention of HIV/AIDS, and postcards with words related to sexual and reproductive rights to send to their friends. In the mixed groups, there was a domination of messages related to HIV/AIDS prevention and sexuality. In groups of females only, messages were more focused on contraceptive methods. A female group developed a 'surprise box' which opened to reveal a penis covered by a condom displaying a message: 'let's take care of each other.' The message used in the 'surprise box' created by a female group was clearly oriented towards men, requesting the use of condoms in order to care for their partners. This strongly expressed the difficulties women experience in convincing men to use condoms. Overall, the usual reference to negotiation skills in relation to condom use and safer sex promotion campaigns is not applicable to the vast majority of women. The cultural barriers faced by women, and especially young girls, are usually far too overpowering to allow them to be in a position to be part of the decision making process with regard to condom use.

In the Northeast, the young people wrote and produced two radio messages that they then recorded with music. They replicated these recorded messages and brought them to local community radios. Out of five texts initially written, they selected two: one about access to contraceptive methods and information about its use, and the other about the myths related to the lack of pleasure when using condoms. A mixed male/female group produced this last message. Females only produced the first one, demonstrating gender differences once again.

In the Northwest, the young people produced two radio commercials, the first being a dialogue in a drugstore between three people buying condoms: a homosexual man, a woman and a heterosexual man. This message focused on the discrimination encountered in relation to sexual preferences and how to avoid it. The second was a dialogue between a father and his teenage daughter about teenage sexuality; the cultural barriers they were facing and how to solve them. This group was composed of young people aged 18 years old and over. Their messages incorporated sexual preference and discrimination, an issue that was not presented by participants in the younger groups from Greater Buenos Aires. The second message clearly expresses the cultural context in which dialogue about sexuality between parents and their children is very unusual.

In the southern area, teenage sexuality was the main issue, focusing on the taboo on discussing sexuality between parents and their sons and daughters. Parents, teachers and adults generally find it difficult to discuss sexuality with adolescents and teenagers. Teenagers presented the words they needed to communicate with adults, showing their difficulty in discussing this with anyone apart from their own age group. In this area, there was less gender difference, possibly because both girls and boys are faced the same difficulties.

Assessment of communication projects

In each area, the final communication products were prepared and tested on a group of 100 young people. In the City of Buenos Aires and in Greater Buenos Aires, these messages were presented to teenagers from secondary schools. Special questionnaires were created in order to compile the opinions of the interviewed teenagers in each area. They were asked to rate each proposal in terms of message, presentation and language in an anonymous survey. Exhibition of the sample results and survey was organized by REDNAC. For the survey, meetings of approximately 20 adolescents were organized in each area, with a suggested total of 100 interviews in each area.

The poster and the 'surprise box' were tested in the City of Buenos Aires with the participation of 60 girls and 40 boys aged between 15 and 17 years old. Both products were received well, respectively considered very good and good (97%). Some 84% of the females and 87% of the males preferred the 'surprise box' which they considered to be more original and attractive. However, a larger proportion of females than males considered its information value to be less significant than that of the posters. We suggest that this is linked to the need of women to convince men to use condoms. The wording was considered good by women and very good by men, especially for being clear and direct. This reflects adolescent's rejection of the adult's habit to use euphemisms or biomedical terminology when discussing issues related to sexuality and reproduction.

In San Miguel, out of 100 people interviewed, 55 were male and 45 female. Both males and females considered the posters to be very good (75% and 70% respectively) and (28% and 21%) as good. There was no gender difference in terms of preference. The highest rating was given to the content of the information (55% of the girls and 63% of the boys), and also the wording was in majority rated as good by both. The design was less appreciated, we believe due to the lack of attractive designs or colours. Overall, they rated the products as good, indicating that content is considered more important than design.

In the Northeast, 100 teenagers were contacted, 65 of which were female and 35 male. Out of the two radio messages assessed, only four girls and one boy considered them to be average and none to be bad. It is interesting to point out that the boys unanimously preferred the focus of promotion of condom use to be directed at HIV/AIDS prevention. The girls were divided equally on their preference for this message and that on myths related to contraception. The gender slant is clear and obvious, as no boy selected the message on forms of contraception, which again confirms the cultural gender pattern that considers contraception to be a women's issue. In this group, too, content was considered most important.

In the Northeast, only 61 young people were surveyed, 41 girls and 20 boys. Some 64% of girls and 57% of boys considered the two radio messages very good. Boys tended to prefer the message with the father-daughter dialogue. Girls, on the other hand, opted most frequently for the question of condom purchase in pharmacies by people with different sexual tendencies. The choice suggests that young men identify with this message because of the presence of the father figure in the dialogue. This raises the issue that boys probably feel frustrated that despite needing to communicate with their fathers on this issue, they often feel that they cannot. This is further supported by previous studies carried out by FEIM that show that these issues are discussed with mothers rather than with fathers (Pagani 2002).

Finally, in the southern area, 61 adolescents were interviewed and there was also a strong female domination: two girls for each boy. In this area, however, although the majority of the participants still rated the messages as good, the proportion of 'very good' recorded was much lower than in the other areas. Some 17% of the girls and 23% of boys considered them to be 'average'. This difference could be due to the age difference (average three years) between the designers of the message and the receivers of the message, indicating that they probably do not relate to them as well. The majority (70% and 72%) of girls and boys preferred the message about sexuality and sexual preference. As in other regions, content of the information was deemed more important than other criteria such as design.

In brief, the validation of the messages in the four areas seems to indicate the need for information. This supersedes the aesthetic quality and the form of presentation, with a few differences in opinion between males and females, that confirm the gender cultural pattern in the country.

Comparison between adults and adolescents

There are noticeable differences between what teenagers think, need and suggest in comparison with adults. One of the messages developed in Greater Buenos Aires revealed one of the main differences. This is the poster showing a male/female couple walking to the health centre with a text: 'We are more responsible than adults think. That's why we want information on how to take care of ourselves when we have sexual relations.' This message alludes to the reproach made by teenagers that the right to information and reproductive health services is denied to them, and includes the accusation of irresponsibility of adults in this issue. As Manangelli and Tejo (2005) have noted, the recognition of adolescents as sexual and reproductive rights subjects is still a bone of contention in Argentina.

The other messages also refer to various claims made by teenagers and denial of their rights, for instance: 'to be given condoms', 'to receive contraceptives in health centres', 'to be able to choose when and with whom to have sexual relations', ' to be able to be a mother or father when they want' and 'not to be forced into starting to be sexually active.' The teenage groups were made up of adolescents under the age of 17, mostly aged between 14 and 15. At 14 and 15, young people face large difficulties in being informed, attended to and provided with contraceptives while, at the same time, they face social pressure to start being sexually active. Young people also want to make informed choices about parenthood and to be able to separate sexual relations from parenthood, requiring the use of and free access to contraceptives. Although this right is established by National Law since October 2002, it still often not enacted because of resistance from the health service and particularly its providers: doctors, nurses and other health personnel.

In the southern area one message was: 'Don't be ashamed to speak out about sexuality, attend the health centre, call us.' The other message was about a dialogue between two teenagers about sexual relations without protection from pregnancy or sexually transmitted infections. This expresses the request of adolescents to receive sexual education in schools, to be allowed to speak about sexuality, sexual and reproductive rights and health, and to demand the right to use and receive contraceptives freely in health care services. While adults considered that young people need to receive information about what to do or what not to do, young people themselves request information to make informed choices. This is based on the Convention on the Rights of the Children, included in Argentinean Constitution since 1994. This seems to be the most important difference that needs to be solved between adults, decision makers and adolescents.

The adolescents and young people request their sexual and reproductive rights to be guaranteed, clearly expressed by all messages and confirmed by the adolescents and young people interviewed. Girls are faced with a double discrimination in these rights, due to their age and gender; boys suffer in general only because of their age. The request to stop discrimination of adolescents and young people in general was also covered in all messages and agreed to by most of the interviewees.

Discussion

In Argentina there are gender and cultural values which make it difficult to address and discuss sexual matters openly. This is particularly the case for adolescents and teenagers, and especially young women. This has a negative biological, psychological and social impact on the health and welfare of young people and particularly young women, as is shown in a persistent increase of adolescent pregnancy rates especially among girls under 15 years of age. In 2002 for the first time, maternal death was registered in this age group.

Last year the national figures showed an increase in HIV/AIDS infection among the population between 15-24 years of age. There is a male-female ratio of 0.8 : 1 in infections in the group aged 15-19 years, indicating the need for skills to empower girls to negotiate condom use. Both government and society need to address this problem if they want to control the HIV/AIDS epidemic in the female adolescent population. A study carried out by FEIM in 2002 predicted this trend (Bianco et al 2003) but now there is evidence to support this. While condom promotion activities are being developed, messages and policies targeting young women and girls for HIV/AIDS prevention are still lacking. The increase of poverty mentioned in the introduction aggravates the HIV/AIDS vulnerability of women and girls: sexual violence has increased, as has sex work or prostitution, both among girls and women and among boys. Prostitution as a survival strategy of families has increased since 2002.

Religious and political conservative groups still oppose sex education in schools and the provision of sexual and reproductive health services to adolescents and young people. This is more evident in the northern areas of the country where the opposition of the community and government is more severe. Because of poverty, secondary school enrolment has dropped to 77.2%. Thus, sexual education needs to be started in primary schools (97.1% enrolment), while strategies have to be developed to reach out-of-school young people.

Notes

The author acknowledges with thanks the help of Josephine LeClerq in the translation of this paper.

References

Bianco, M., 'Fertility, health and poverty in Latin America: the Argentinian case'. Buenos Aires, Fundación para Estudio e Investigación de la Mujer (FEIM) and United Nations Population Fund (UNFPA), 1996.

Bianco, M. et al, 'Adolescence in Argentina: sexuality and poverty'. Buenos Aires, Fundación para Estudio e Investigación de la Mujer (FEIM) and United Nations Population Fund (UNFPA), 2003.

Manangelli, S. and M.T. Tejo, 'Sexual and reproductive rights: an approach to the discourse in Argentinian news papers'. Thesis for the Communication School, University of Buenos Aires, 2005.

Pagani, L. et al, 'Adolescents, sexual and reproductive rights and health policies in Buenos Aires City'. *DeSIDAmos* vol. 10, no. 1 (2002), p. 25-29.

gender and health: policy and practice

4 Men, gender equity and HIV/AIDS prevention, with case studies from South Africa and Brazil

At a seminar at New York City's public library a few years ago, André de Zanger of the Creativity Institute mesmerized his audience by discussing a Soviet-devised problem-solving model called the Theory of Inventive Problem Solving, otherwise known as TRIZ. TRIZ, developed in a resource-poor nation, invites practitioners to invent new ways of using limited resources to solve problems. It encourages analysts and inventors to look for obvious but often hidden solutions within existing systems and structures. The management adage – the problem is part of the solution and the solution is part of the problem – encapsulates the TRIZ approach (Altshuller 1994).

One can begin applying TRIZ, says de Zanger, by imagining how people, and existing tools and equipment, might be used outside their normative functions. How can current functions be converted to create an entirely new system or machine? Several years ago, for example, the beverage industry found that their cans for fruit juices and fizzy drinks were collapsing during shipping, resulting in millions of dollars of lost sales. The industry was confronted with a need to make a stronger can without adding significant extra costs. With minimal expense, they fortified their aluminium cans by adding more nitrogen gas to the liquid *inside* the can rather than tinkering with its external structure (Altshuller 1994). TRIZ has a proven track record in manufacturing and industry, bringing innovation and huge cost savings to companies like Thales, Rolls Royce, Boeing and BAE Systems (Beeby 2005). Some commentators, like de Zanger, believe it may also be possible to apply it to social and political problems as well. How, for example, might TRIZ principles be applied to global efforts to prevent HIV/AIDS infections?

The HIV and gender violence prevention projects highlighted in this paper reflect a new and growing type of intervention in the fight against HIV/AIDS; one that focuses on men and boys as allies actively engaged in efforts to promote women's rights and to expand effective and equitable reproductive health for men and women. The two case studies from South Africa and Brazil illustrate the use of TRIZ, looking at the involvement of men and boys and the roles they can play in HIV and gender violence prevention.

HIV prevention and TRIZ

TRIZ may provide a useful approach to HIV prevention in resource-poor regions of the world. Sub-Saharan Africa, Asia, Eastern Europe and the former USSR all share common traits of chronic poverty, and poor health and social service infrastructure.

Today, the vast majority of HIV/AIDS cases, approximately 90%, are found in sub-Saharan Africa.

In the USA, the Mentors in Violence Prevention Strategies, Inc. (MVP) employed TRIZ-style principles in a number of its projects. MVP's pedagogy explicitly calls for male facilitators to interact with male participants as *bystanders* who have the potential to interrupt violence rather than as potential *perpetrators* who have the power to harm women. Using a teaching technique that does not blame or shame men, MVP has attracted hundreds of thousands of men and boys to work against gender violence in the last 15 years. It has established programmes and networks in the US Marine Corps and Navy, high schools, colleges and communities. It has also succeeded in opening new dialogue and partnerships between pro-feminist men and boys and female veterans of the battered women's movement globally. Jackson Katz, director of MVP, believes this same approach can be applied to HIV prevention, relying on men and boys' responsibility to themselves and family and community as a point of entry:

> There is a reason why men have not been speaking out about AIDS prevention, speaking out about men's responsibility on this subject. There are large numbers of men invested in a certain definition of manhood that keeps the current system in place, that is to say, sexual inequality, the subordinate position of women, the pressures to have multiple partners. If this is the case, then reframing the conversation of HIV prevention as a men's issue and directly challenging cultural definitions of manhood is a key strategy for change...we are challenging deeply seated ideas about manhood. That is why we face so much resistance. We need much more public honesty among men. Many men are trained to present themselves as invulnerable, especially men in leadership. Somehow any hint of our weaknesses, our mistakes, is a demonstration of our lack of power or authority. Some of the best leadership comes from men who admit they are not perfect. (Zoll 2004c)

An important step in the TRIZ process is forming 'a new system that unites objects in such a way that a new feature appears' (Altshuller 1994). Could it be that a powerful new feature for reducing heterosexual HIV transmission might be found within the context of heterosexual transmission itself? Might the overlooked and underutilized resources in current HIV prevention work be the very men and boys who do care and respect the women in their lives, and who desperately want to protect them from infection?

Such a suggestion does not always fall easily on the ears of seasoned veterans within the field of international development. Discussions about funding programmes specifically for men and boys are often perceived as a direct strike against the already limited funding mechanisms earmarked for women and girls. Given the slow history of integrating any kind of substantial gender analysis and equity goals into development objectives, women's advocates have a legitimate reason to feel threatened.

It was only a decade ago in 1994 that decision makers at the International Conference on Population and Development in Cairo, Egypt, agreed to make women the centrepiece of a new development paradigm. At this historic gathering, the international community agreed that targeting resources at women was more likely to lift families out of poverty and sustain basic development goals, such as education, health care and nutrition. From Cairo, a new language came into being, including 'gender mainstreaming' and new strategies for integrating gender equity into all levels of development, not just the typically under-funded and under-staffed women's divisions and agencies.

While the Cairo paradigm proved successful in a vast number of development scenarios, the AIDS pandemic has drastically offset goals in poverty alleviation, maternal and child health, girls' education, and access to health care. At this point of time in the evolution of the HIV/AIDS pandemic in which infection accelerates via male-to-female transmission, another paradigm may need to be invented and implemented. This time, it may need to focus more intensely on men and boys as agents of dramatic intervention.

Increased female HIV/AIDS infection

Patterns of HIV/AIDS infection vary from country to country. Information provided by the Joint United Nations Programme on HIV/AIDS (UNAIDS) shows that dirty needles, contaminated blood and men having sex with men continue to pose serious risks of HIV infection globally. Heterosexual sex, however, appears to be the fastest growing route of infection today, particularly among women (UNAIDS et al 2004). UNAIDS has reported a trend of higher infections among young women aged 15-24 in many regions of Africa, and some areas of Asia and Eastern Europe. In Zambia, Zimbabwe and South Africa, the number of infections among 15-24 year old girls and young women is four to six times higher than their male peers (Quinn 2005).

According to the UNAIDS 2004 'Global report on the HIV/AIDS epidemic':
- In sub-Saharan Africa an estimated 25 million people are HIV positive. Of these, 57% of infected adults are women and 75% of infected young people are women and girls between the ages of 15 and 24. Many equate these high numbers of female infection to extreme poverty among women and poor enforcement of women's human, economic and educational rights.
- In China, as many as 10 million people may be infected by 2010. Public health officials have tracked early HIV infections to tainted blood transfusions in poor rural areas but injecting drug use is also fuelling transmission. Today heterosexual transmission is escalating, particularly among women.
- The Russian Federation has the largest number of people living with HIV in the region, estimated at 860,000 (range: 420 000-1.4 million). During the last ten years, economic and political upheaval in the former USSR has created a black market economy that has reduced the cost of heroine to that of a bottle of Coca-Cola, making it that much easier for frustrated, unemployed young men to buy (Zoll 2003a). Male intravenous drug users under the age of 30 were the first demographic group to register HIV-positive but transmission is now spreading fastest among their female sexual partners.
- India has the largest number of people living with HIV outside South Africa, estimated at 4.6 million in 2002. Most infections are thought to be acquired through heterosexual sex, while a small proportion is acquired through injecting drug use.

From this growing rate of increased female infection globally, we may conclude that many HIV prevention strategies are not protecting women and girls, and most are likely not challenging the inequitable gender norms that increase women and girls level of risk of infection.

Gender roles

The inequalities and dysfunctions of contemporary male-female gender roles and power dynamics lie at the heart of the HIV/AIDS pandemic. With women and girls becoming infected more often than men, it is imperative that prevention initiatives begin to integrate gender-sensitive perspectives into overall school-based and community prevention education programmes (Barroso 2005). At the 13th International AIDS Conference in Durban, South Africa, Geeta Rao Gupta of the International Center for Research on Women (ICRW), based in Washington DC, discussed the issue of power between men and women engaged in heterosexual relationships:

> *Power is fundamental to both sexuality and gender. The unequal power balance in gender relations that favours men, translates into an unequal power balance in heterosexual interactions, in which male pleasure supersedes female pleasure and men have greater control than women over when, where, and how sex takes place. An understanding of individual sexual behaviour, male or female, thus, necessitates an understanding of gender and sexuality as constructed by a complex interplay of social, cultural, and economic forces that determine the distribution of power. Research supported by ICRW and conducted by researchers worldwide has identified the different ways in which the imbalance in power between women and men in gender relations curtails women's sexual autonomy and expands male sexual freedom, thereby increasing women AND men's risk and vulnerability to HIV.*
> (Gupta 2000)

Gender research conducted over the last 20 years in Latin America, Asia and Africa reveals that despite social, cultural and religious differences, there are many universally shared beliefs about how men and women should behave socially and sexually. For men, this might include pursuing sexual relations with multiple partners, engaging in unprotected sex, and ignoring important reproductive health and general health needs (International HIV/AIDS Alliance 2003).

- In Guatemala, research conducted in 1996 revealed a widely held perception among males *and* females that having numerous sexual partners was a necessary feature of young men's physical and mental development (Weiss et al 1996).
- In Nicaragua, where virginity is highly valued among young women, having multiple sexual partners is taken as a sign of virility in young men. Teenage boys face social pressures from older men, including fathers, older brothers and uncles, to have sex as early as possible. In the recent past, it was not uncommon for fathers to arrange for their son's sexual initiation with a sex worker (Zelaya et al 1997). For many young Nicaraguan men, the pressure to be sexually active and multi-partnered may be so great that those who do not fulfil this expectation are open to ridicule by their peers for not being a 'real man' (Rivers and Aggleton 1999).

- In Thailand, 15 year-old boys are not considered 'real men' until they have visited a commercial sex worker (Hata 1995).

In many regions of the world, men and boys place themselves and their partners at risk by ignoring their health needs and shunning available prevention and health care services (Hata 1995). Though HIV-positive men do not appear to suffer social stigma as severely as women and girls, many report that they are afraid to access services for fear of public humiliation or individual fears about the disease and its effect on their lives. In addition, men and boys are socially expected to be able to endure pain. Research shows that rather than seeking appropriate care, males tend often to self medicate with alcohol, substance abuse or risky behaviours, including sexual behaviours (Keijzer et al 2001).

Women and girls, on the other hand, are expected to remain passive and ignorant in the arena of sexuality (Gupta 2000), and to accept their subordinate position to men and boys. These social expectations, coupled with poor enforcement of women's human and economic rights, extreme poverty and illiteracy, greatly increase women and girl's risk of contracting HIV (UNAIDS et al 2004).

- In Zambia, a study by the World YWCA indicated that fewer than 25% of women believed a wife could refuse sex with her husband. Only 11% believed she had a right to ask him to use a condom (2002).
- In Zimbabwe, male and female high school students believed boys should have many girlfriends while girls should have only one boyfriend (UNAIDS 1999).

Given these examples, one might conclude that adolescents need much greater access to more gender-sensitive HIV prevention approaches. Jill Lewis is the co-founder of the Nordic Living for Tomorrow Project, a UNAIDS Best Practice gender-sensitive HIV prevention programme. For the last 20 years, Lewis has been conducting HIV prevention and gender training with educators and health care providers in Africa, Asia and Europe. One of the fundamental components of her successful training module has been facilitating open discourse between male and female participants about the ways in which gender roles and behaviours have and continue to change over time (Lewis 2001). She considers that:

> The ability to change is proof that gender systems are not fixed points in any one culture or religious system. (Zoll 2003a)

The fact that most HIV prevention programmes do not integrate or operate from a gender-sensitive perspective is an indication of how many populations are accepting these roles as 'normal' or 'natural'. The notion that there is a 'natural and innate gender order' essentially silences efforts to talk about it, says Lewis.

There are more than three billion young people and children in the world today who are or will become sexually active in the very near future (UNFPA undated). These young adults are the most vulnerable to HIV infection. Many have little or no access to HIV prevention materials, condoms or public forums where they can comfortably discuss gender and sexuality (Zoll 2003b). Yet it is this same population that is the most likely to adopt new sexual behaviours and attitudes that can promote gender equity rather than perpetuate gender inequality. Perhaps as a result of witnessing the deaths of parents, siblings, relatives and friends, these young men and women are being forced out of a need for survival to re-evaluate how they communicate about and behave sexually, and how they interact with the opposite sex. Such endeavours may save their lives (Zoll 2004a).

Men and HIV prevention

In 2003, the International HIV/AIDS Alliance with support from the US Agency for International Development (USAID) surveyed dozens of HIV/AIDS programmes in all regions of the world specifically working with men and boys to curb the pandemic and to reduce gender violence. The report highlights 13 case studies in Morocco, Botswana, Bangladesh, South Africa, Mongolia, Pakistan, India, Zambia and Belarus (International HIV/AIDS Alliance 2003).

With a focus on sexual health and reproductive responsibility linked to HIV and gender violence prevention, these programmes support women and men's rights in the following manner:
- Working on behalf of both women and men's right to access health care services, with strong emphasis on shifting men's attitudes about avoidance of health care. This work reframes health care as a man's issue, enabling men and boys to feel more comfortable seeking care.
- Encouraging men's support of women's human rights by reframing manhood to no longer equate manliness with domination over women and girls.
- Promoting health and human rights by improving understanding about relationship dynamics between heterosexual partners and creating a healthier environment for families.

This important publication highlights the accelerating growth of the global men's health movement. A major theme among the featured programmes was men's increasing willingness to explore and examine their own and socially dictated attitudes and behaviours about manhood and masculinity. The report, and subsequent regional and global conferences, has further solidified this grassroots movement's credibility, and done much to forge stronger alliances between women and men's organizations dedicated to gender equity and universal human rights (Zoll 2004b).

A majority of these programmes provide men and boys with gender-equitable male role models to help them redefine manhood and manliness in ways that do not equate masculinity with aggression and domination (Barker 2000). With a goal of deconstructing masculinities, male programme leaders often encourage boys and men to examine their behaviour in relation to women, to assume greater sexual and reproductive health responsibility, including HIV prevention, and to help end gender violence. While this kind of approach to HIV prevention is still somewhat rare (Zoll 2003a), many male activists have successfully used the deconstruction model in programmes aimed at reducing domestic and sexual violence (Zoll 2004c). In South Africa, for example, men are calling upon the same men who helped tear down apartheid to interrupt the twin epidemics of HIV/AIDS and high rates of men's violence against women. Since 1997, the South African government and NGOs have helped organize men's marches, or *imbizos*, to mobilize massive community involvement in gender violence and HIV prevention efforts (South African Press Association 2002).

Case study: Men as Partners, South Africa

In South Africa, the Men as Partners (MaP) project is challenging men and women's perspectives about gender roles and behaviours that elevate HIV infection. A project of Planned Parenthood South Africa and EngenderHealth, MaP is specifically working to reduce HIV/AIDS transmission and men's epidemic violence against women. The programme's ambitious goals include reaching more than 60,000 members of the South African Defence Force, 800,000 male union members and hundreds of thousands of men and boys involved in a vast network of HIV/AIDS organizations nationally (Peacock undated).

Dean Peacock, a MaP programme manager and technical advisor, came to the HIV prevention movement through gender violence prevention work in the USA. Based on his work with men who are violent with their female partners, Peacock says he realized how essential it was to create safe environments where men and boys could investigate and discuss gender roles, sexism, violence, and HIV prevention (Zoll 2003c). Peacock has found that men in the USA and South Africa, rich or poor, are 'very open to gender equitable work' (Zoll 2003c):

> The paradox about the [HIV/AIDS] epidemic is that is has opened the door to gender equality. We are certainly not three generations away from men playing a leadership role in HIV prevention and violence prevention. This notion that there is a monolithic African male who manifests all of these negative stereotypes is reactionary. Masculinity in all cultures is much more dynamic and fluid. I was recently at training sponsored by the Commonwealth and was amazed by the men in the room. They were senior members of parliament, and many of them were doctors. They were all able to articulate the issues clearly, and they are the men in their 50s and 60s who some say are resisting this paradigm change that can shift men from being part of the problem to being part of the solution.

Patrick Godana is a MaP graduate and trainer in the Eastern Cape who works with male truck drivers, one of the highest HIV risk groups. In Africa, as elsewhere in the developing world where poverty and gender inequality is pervasive, truck stops are often filled with young girls and women selling sex in exchange for money, food or other essentials. Godana says many of the drivers have told him it is 'manly' for them to have extramarital affairs while they are away from their families. In order to confront the dangers to which men were exposing themselves, Godana organized focus groups where the men could talk freely about fellow drivers who had died from AIDS and about condoms:

You know, those guys never actually understood what a condom is. Some of them say it is a poison [that] it is from the whites who do not want us to have children. One actually has to go and listen to them and to try and interact and challenge them and let them open up so you can give them informed information. I say to them, "In any kind of work there are overalls, and this kind of work you are doing, you must use condoms as overalls and protect yourself as well so as to live longer." (Peacock 2001)

Like Godana, Steven Ngobeni participated in MaP trainings and found himself challenging entrenched male peer culture and gender roles in his village. Despite difficult conversations and ridicule from both men and women, he eventually succeeded in shifting long-held beliefs about the division of labour based on gender (Peacock 2001). Shortly after his marriage, Ngobeni came face-to-face with the unfair burden of domestic chores his new wife was forced to attend to on a daily basis simply because she was a woman:

What was expected from my wife was for her to wake up early in the morning – before I could even wake up – to sweep outside and prepare everything herself, you see, for the entire family. Just because she is the wife, it is what she is expected to do. They want to see this woman go to the veld and fetch that firewood, and come back with that firewood on her head. It is a very challenging situation.

In the village, the women have to carry water five kilometres. It was really working on me so I said that we must put money, each man, so we can hire men with pick-up trucks to take them water. Everyone was so angry with me, saying that I am collaborating, that the women have talked to me, that these women are sitting here doing nothing. If you look at our muscles they are big and we can carry that, but we say the women must carry.

So I challenged that and it changed my home. No more are the women carrying big buckets. We arranged to hire somebody and we have pick-ups. Why not take this truck and get in the back and ask the young man to get some water? Basically they say it is our tradition and culture that women must bring this water. But the water is the same. They drink the same water. So it is very challenging for me as a person to change the system. (Peacock 2003)

In the context of the HIV/AIDS pandemic, Ngobeni's actions probably had far-reaching positive effects on the women in his village.

Throughout the entire Southern Africa region, governments and donors are relying on communities to provide care and support to those infected and affected by the pandemic. Women and girls comprise the backbone of these unpaid care networks, juggling the majority of care for millions of orphans and people living with the virus (Zoll 2005). According to the UN Development Fund for Women (UNIFEM), an AIDS patient in Zimbabwe requires an estimated 24 buckets of water per day (Heyzer 2002). Some of this is used for cooking, some for constant cleaning, laundry and bathing of those who are sick or dying from AIDS, or for millions of children made vulnerable or orphaned as a result of the pandemic. The job of hauling water can take anywhere from four to six hours a day or longer, depending on the distance from a village to a water well. Studies in Burkina Faso, Uganda and Zambia indicate that women and girls could save hundreds of hours a year if walking to sources of fuelwood and water were reduced to 30 minutes or less (UNDP undated).

Ngobeni's decision to organize men to hire a truck was an exceptional example of TRIZ in action. By utilizing one tool – the truck – he was able to offset rigid gender roles and to solve a time and labour burden thereby creating more 'free' time for the girls and women in his village. Although there has been no formal follow-up to Ngobeni's actions, it is likely that some girls in his village were able to return to school during the same hours they used to spend hauling water. It is also possible that some women who were forced to quit paid employment in order to care for the sick or orphaned may have returned to work. Both education and economic autonomy are important strategies for reducing women and girls' risk of HIV infection (UNFPA 2004).

Dynamic male leadership like that demonstrated by Ngobeni is often missing from broader global efforts to promote HIV prevention, gender equity and sexual health responsibility. This is due in part to the very nature of masculinity, its codes and peer pressures, which often interfere with caring men's ability to publicly stand up for women or other men. It also stems from women's historic and often realistic mistrust of men, and women's desire to liberate themselves without assistance from men.

Case study: Instituto Promundo, Brazil

In the busy streets of Rio de Janeiro, the staff at Instituto Promundo (IP) are studying how young boys and men are socialized, and how their peer culture influences behaviours that put them at risk to HIV infection. Since 1998, IP's gender, health and adolescence programmes have involved young men in the promotion of responsible health care and gender equity in intimate and professional relationships with women and girls. Reaching more than 1500 men annually, IP works in collaboration and partnership with ECOS, an NGO in Sao Paulo, PAPAI in Recife, and Salud y Genero in Mexico. It also works with the Pan American Health Organization and the International Planned Parenthood Federation (John Snow Inc 2005).

IP's community condom campaign, *Hora H*, is situated in a low-income suburb in the western stretches of Bangu, a population of 600,000, comprised mostly of low-income and working class families. With support from Durex Condoms, Europe's largest condom distributor, IP asked boys aged 15-22 for their ideas on how they would move condoms out into the community among their peers (Barker undated). The boys came up with the idea of the *Hora H* brand condom, which translates from the Portuguese into English as: 'In the heat of the moment.'

While IP's primary goals strive for HIV and gender violence prevention, it is equally committed to building a gender equitable generation among the young men and women in Rio de Janeiro, and throughout Brazil and the world. The success of the *Hora H* campaign is being measured not only through condom sales and distribution to peers in the neighbourhood. It is also being measured by how equitably the young men and women in the community treat one another (Barker undated).

men, gender equity and hiv/aids prevention

73

Rooted in the idea of promoting a lifestyle among young men that enables them to care for their own sexual health and that of their partners, the condom is used as a way of marketing gender equitable behaviours and attitudes. In the case of young men, according to Gary Barker and Marcos Nascimento who direct and conduct research at IP, condom use is one of the factors highly associated with gender equitable behaviour. Whether a young man uses a condom depends on whether he buys into traditional notions of masculinity or not (Barker 2000). In his research, Barker has found that young men less attached to traditional ideas of masculinity were more likely to use condoms and less likely to engage in violence against women (Barker 2000). As Zoll notes:

> The young men who were more rigid in their gender identification did not use condoms as often, and were more likely to feel entitled about engaging in sexual relations with multiple partners. Young people's sexual activity is driven by social norms and peer culture. IP's focus on young men and HIV prevention revolves around the question of: how do you build condom use into the idea of building a gender equitable lifestyle that young men, and women, can embrace? (Zoll 2004d)

IP's qualitative research has found more gender equitable behaviours among men and boys who have reflected about the costs of traditional versions of masculinity, either alone or in a group. According to Barker's 1999 research study, 'Gender equitable boys in a gender equitable world' (Barker 2000), young men and women need a physical space or some kind of social structure where they can evaluate and discuss what these costs have meant to them personally. This kind of social structure and peer group support enables non-traditional behaviours to flourish in a safe environment. In Malawi, Save the Children, CARE and UN agencies have put this theory to work by sponsoring Girls Clubs and Youth Clubs that revolve around teaching young people life skills, including HIV prevention and male-female gender roles (USAID et al 2004).

Conclusions

The HIV prevention projects highlighted here reflect a new and growing type of intervention in the fight against HIV/AIDS. Partially as a result of witnessing the HIV/AIDS pandemic, a new generation of pro-feminist men is challenging entrenched gender norms and behaviours that contribute to infection and violence against women. This kind of visible male leadership is directly and indirectly granting permission to thousands of boys and young men in all regions of the world to redefine and question ideas and perceptions of masculinities. The growth of the global men's health movement, and the integration of gender-sensitive perspectives into HIV prevention strategies, is one positive outcome of the HIV/AIDS pandemic. Initiatives such as Men as Partners and *Hora H* are providing men and boys with new opportunities to redefine what it means to be a man in the age of AIDS. This new framework is creating enormous opportunities for activists from around the world to call upon men and boys to demonstrate leadership where little male leadership until now may have been demonstrated.

The absence of a gender equitable peer network, as demonstrated by the Brazilian case study, makes it difficult for men and boys to sustain egalitarian behaviours. A young man choosing to be in a monogamous relationship, for example, may be ridiculed by his primary male peer group that pressures him to prove his manhood by engaging with multiple sexual partners. This same peer policing dynamic was visible in the South African village where Steven Ngobeni proposed hiring a truck to haul water. When he first proposed the idea, the men teased him and accused him of collaborating with the women.

Sexually active young people between the ages of 15 and 24, and children orphaned by AIDS, are most vulnerable to HIV/AIDS infection, particularly young women in sub-Saharan Africa, a region steeped in gender inequality, economic deprivation and poor quality and delivery of health services. While they are most at risk, this young population is also most likely to become aware of and adopt new gendered sexual behaviours and attitudes that embody greater equality between women and men.

Until now, prescribed gender roles in almost every culture have encouraged men to dominate and women to appear passive, not only in sexual relations but in the world at large. The fulfilment of women and girls' human and economic rights is a central building block in curbing the spread of HIV/AIDS. Expanding attention and greater funds toward men's participation in HIV/AIDS prevention and sexual and reproductive health programmes will probably accelerate efforts to meet these important gender equity goals.

References

Altshuller, Genrich (H. Altov), 'And suddenly the inventor appeared: TRIZ, the theory of inventive problem solving'. Translated by Lev Shulyak. Worcester, MA, Technical Innovation Center, 1994.

Barroso, Carmen, 'Gender, youth and AIDS.' Paper presented at 'Achievements, gaps and challenges in linking the implementation of the Beijing Platform for Action and the Millennium Declaration and Millennium Development Goals', Baku, Azerbaijan, 7-10 February 2005.

Barker, Gary, 'Gender equitable boys in a gender equitable world: reflections from qualitative research and program development with young men in Rio de Janeiro'. *Sexual and Relationship Therapy* vol. 15, no. 3 (2000), p. 263-282.

Barker, Gary, 'Instituto PROMUNDO: engaging young men in gender-based violence prevention and sexual and reproductive health promotion'. Rio de Janeiro, Instituto PROMUNDO, undated.

Beeby, Heather, 'TRIZ for the aerospace industry: an introduction to creative problem solving'. London, IBM UK, 2005.

Gupta, Geeta Rao, 'Gender, sexuality and HIV/AIDS: the what, the why and the how'. Plenary address, XIIIth International AIDS Conference, Durban, South Africa, July 12, 2000.

Hata, P.U., 'We must be a caring society, not a scared society'. In: E. Reid (ed.), *HIV & AIDS: the global inter-connection*. Bloomfield, CT, Kumarian Press, 1995.

Heyzer, Noeleen, 'The unequal AIDS burden'. *Christian Science Monitor* July 18 (2002).

International HIV/AIDS Alliance, 'Working with men, responding to AIDS. Gender, sexuality and HIV/AIDS: a case study collection'. Brighton, International HIV/AIDS Alliance, 2003.

John Snow Inc. and JSI Research and Training Institute, Inc., 'Project M: promoting young women's empowerment and sexual and reproductive health in Brazil'. Boston, MA, John Snow, Inc, 2005.

Keijzer, B. de, E.M. Reyes, O. Aguilar, G. Sanchez, and G. Ayala, 'Working with men on gender, health and violence'. Mexico, December 2001.

Lewis, Jill, 'Mobilizing gender issues'. *NIKK Magazine* no. 3 (2001), p. 19-21.

Peacock, Dean, 'Building on a legacy of social justice activism: enlisting men as gender justice activists in South Africa'. *Men and Masculinities* vol. 5, no. 3 (2003), p. 325-328.

Peacock, Dean, 'Men as Partners: South African men respond to violence against women and HIV/AIDS'. New York, NY, EngenderHealth, undated.

Peacock, Dean, 'The Men as Partners Programme: working with men in Southern Africa to end violence against and prevent HIV/AIDS'. Johannesburg, November 2001.

Quinn, Thomas C., 'Johns Hopkins AIDS expert says global strategy needed to combat "feminization" of HIV/AIDS'. Baltimore, MD, Johns Hopkins Medicine, June 2005.

Rivers, K. and P. Aggleton, 'Adolescent sexuality, gender and the HIV epidemic'. New York, NY, United Nations Development Programme (UNDP), 1999.

South African Press Association, 'Concerted effort needed to combat spread of HIV/AIDS: Zuma'. Johannesburg, South African Press Association, October 2002.

UNAIDS, 'Gender and HIV/AIDS: taking stock of research and programmes'. Geneva, Joint United Nations Programme on HIV/AIDS (UNAIDS), 1999.

UNAIDS, UNFPA and UNIFEM, 'Women and HIV/AIDS: confronting the crisis'. Geneva and New York NY, Joint United Nations Programme on HIV/AIDS (UNAIDS), United Nations Population Fund (UNFPA) and United Nations Development Fund for Women (UNIFEM), 2004.

UNDP, 'Frameworks for action, biodiversity and the Millennium Development Goals'. Washington, DC, United Nations Development Programme (UNDP), undated at http://www.undp.org

UNFPA, 'State of world population 2004. The Cairo consensus at ten: population, reproductive health and the global effort to end poverty'. New York, NY, United Nations Population Fund (UNFPA), 2004

UNFPA, 'Supporting adolescents and youth. Investing in adolescents and youth can yield wide ranging dividends'. New York, NY, United Nations Population Fund (UNFPA), undated.

USAID, UNICEF, UNAIDS, WFP-Policy Project-Futures Group International, 'OVC RAAAP Malawi Country Report'. Washington, DC, United States Agency for International Development (USAID), United Nations Children's Fund (UNICEF), Joint United Nations Programme on HIV/AIDS (UNAIDS), WFP-Policy Project-Futures Group International, 2004.

Weiss, E., D. Whelan, and G. Gupta, 'Vulnerability and opportunity: adolescents and HIV/AIDS in the developing world'. Washington, DC, International Center for Research on Women (ICRW), 1996.

World YWCA, 'Our call to lead: AIDS in the developing world'. Geneva, World Young Women's Christian Association (YWCA), 2002.

Zelaya, E., F.M. Marín, J. García, S. Berglund, J. Liljestrand, and L.A. Persson, 'Gender and social differences in adolescent sexuality and reproduction in Nicaragua'. *Journal of Adolescent Health* vol. 21, no. 1 (1997), p. 39-46.

Zoll, Miriam, 'Draft Joint UN Agency Publication on 'Women and HIV/AIDS: confronting the crisis'. Geneva and New York, NY, Joint United Nations Programme on HIV/AIDS (UNAIDS), United Nations Population Fund (UNFPA), United Nations Fund for Women (UNIFEM), 2004a.

Zoll, Miriam, Interview with Jill Lewis, Living for Tomorrow Program, for joint UN Agency publication on 'Women and HIV/AIDS: confronting the crisis', New York, December 2003a.

Zoll, Miriam, Interview with Alice Welbourne, Living for Tomorrow Program, for joint UN Agency publication on 'Women and HIV/AIDS: confronting the crisis', New York, NY, December 2003b.

Zoll, Miriam, Interview with Dean Peacock, Men as Partners, for Joint UN Agency Publication on 'Women and HIV/AIDS: confronting the crisis', New York, NY, December 2003c.

Zoll, Miriam, Interview with Dean Peacock, Men as Partners, for Joint UN Agency Publication on 'Women and HIV/AIDS: confronting the crisis', New York, NY, March 2004b.

Zoll, Miriam, Interview with Gary Barker for Joint UN Agency publication on 'Women and HIV/AIDS: confronting the crisis, New York, NY, 2004d.

oll, Miriam, Interview with Jackson Katz, Founder, Mentors in Violence Prevention Program, for Joint UN Agency publication on 'Women and HIV/AIDS: confronting the crisis, New York, NY, 2004c.

oll, Miriam, 'Executive summary: OVC RAAP Initiative final report'. Washington, DC and Geneva, United States Agency for International Development (USAID), United Nations Children's Fund (UNICEF), Joint United Nations Programme on HIV/AIDS (UNAIDS), WFP-Policy Project-Futures Group International, 2005. http://www.futuresgroup.com/ovc

Madeleen Wegelin-Schuringa

5 Local responses to HIV/AIDS from a gender perspective

Between 2002 and 2004, the Royal Tropical Institute (KIT) in Amsterdam has managed the development of a toolkit for local responses to HIV and AIDS for the Joint United Nations Programme on HIV/AIDS (UNAIDS). The aim of the toolkit is to strengthen the capacity of different actors to address HIV/AIDS at local level, to take concrete measures to reduce vulnerability and risk, and to mitigate the impact of the epidemic on affected households and communities.

The process of developing the toolkit started with a workshop with partners from Brazil, Burkina Faso, Trinidad and Tobago, Thailand, Uganda and Zambia to design a framework to document programmes and approaches in such a way that readers could apply the approaches by themselves and adapt them to their own context. On the basis of case studies that the partners brought with them, two frameworks were developed, one for participatory approaches (techniques) and one for programmes (practices). In the next phase, KIT staff visited the countries of the partner institutions to help document ongoing programmes that were identified by the partner institutions. In the documentation process, the staff of these programmes were facilitated to look critically at their own programmes and to analyse the crucial aspects that made the programme successful and the issues that could be improved. In addition to these visits, interesting programmes in other countries were identified and asked to document their programme according to the framework. These programmes were reviewed and commented upon in an iterative process.

This process has resulted in 20 techniques and 50 practices in the toolkit, taken from 14 countries across the world. The toolkit is published by KIT and UNAIDS and is available as an online publication on KIT's website (www.kit.nl/publishers/). Participatory techniques help a facilitator to support an audience to analyse their own situation and to establish their needs and priorities, in order to plan interventions. The practices describe, in a practical way, the process that is carried out by an organization, institution or community to address one or more specific problem, giving an analysis of critical issues and lessons learnt. Each practice can serve as an example and/or inspiration for others that are confronted with a similar problem.

The programmes described in the toolkit show that the combination of empowerment of key actors and multi-sectoral support to their interventions can be effective in developing capacities of local communities to tackle HIV/AIDS issues within their own environment. The way in which individuals, men and women, families and communities behave is of prime importance to effectively address the epidemic. Responses to HIV are thus in the first instance local: they imply the involvement of men and women where they live, namely in their homes, their neighbourhoods and their work places. Although the responses are local, analysis of the techniques and practices in the toolkit reveals that there are a number of common aspects addressing similar problems or similar target groups, be it in a different community or country.

The aim of this paper is to discuss these aspects in order to contribute to further strategy development in local responses to HIV/AIDS, with specific attention to gender implications. The paper is based on an analysis of the programmes that are part of the toolkit and on discussions held with staff of these programmes during the process of documenting the techniques and practices. The aspects covered are prevention through peer education; home-based care; involvement of people living with HIV/AIDS; the role of faith-based organizations; and approaches to increase sharing of knowledge and learning within countries.

Prevention through peer education

The majority of the practices in the toolkit (27 out of 50) deal with prevention, and many focus on awareness raising with different target groups. Peer education is the most common approach and, according to people involved, effective because people prefer to take advice from peers who understand their cultural, social and economic environment rather than from outsiders. Some issues that are common in many of the toolkit programmes are discussed below. These pertain to the methods and motivation of peer educators and the linkages with support services. Monitoring the impact of peer education programmes, discussed as evidence of the effectiveness of peer education programmes, is not strong and many programmes struggle to develop a good monitoring system.

Peer education requires participatory approaches but also linkages to support services

Youth peer education activities make use of participatory methods of awareness raising, life skills education and empowerment. Where drama and role plays are performed, it is the discussion afterwards that leads to more understanding of vulnerability. Such discussions are often held in same sex groups, as vulnerabilities of male and female youth are different and require different strategies. The participatory techniques increase commitment and ownership of interventions to overcome the vulnerability of the target groups.

With the peer educators themselves, involvement in planning and design of communication methods from the start, not only leads to ownership of the peer education activities, but also to a more equal balance between the sexes. This is necessary because male peer educators tend to dominate decision making and only in groups that stay together over a longer period or where females outstay males (which is often the case) do females become sufficiently empowered to take the lead or at least have an equal influence. The youth peer education activities tend to concentrate on awareness raising, life skills and on promotion of condom use. While in all programmes the increase in knowledge about HIV/AIDS, growing understanding of vulnerabilities and increased access to condoms is demonstrated, actual behaviour change is not an automatic outcome.

It is remarkable that only one youth programme actually developed linkages with 'youth friendly services'. This is in Jhapa, Moram and Illam Districts of Nepal (Practice 25) where Save the Children initiated collaboration with organizations providing youth-friendly health and sexually transmitted infection (STI) services to respond to the demand for services by youth, after mobilization by peer educators. This resulted in a 60% increase of visits for STI treatment or counselling in one district clinic.

In adult peer education programmes, the situation is different. These programmes are all linked to support services that are a priority for the target group, such as STI clinics, general health services and legal support, and hence go beyond awareness raising and understanding of vulnerabilities. In addition to these services, the programmes focus on the creation of an enabling environment by involving key organizations of that environment such as the police, brothel owners, drug dealers and truck owners. The adult peer education is mainly carried out with specific target groups of at risk communities such as female sex workers, men having sex with men, intravenous drug users and mobile populations such as truck drivers. Peer educators are selected from these groups according to agreed criteria and interest.

Sustaining motivation of peer educators

The challenge to maintain and motivate interest with unpaid or low paid peer educators pertains to all programmes in the toolkit. Yet, if the main approach in prevention is through peer education, it is essential that strategies to sustain motivation are developed from the start.

Peer educators may become project staff and receive a salary, ensuring sustainability of the peer education intervention at least for the time of the project. However, in most cases, the trained peer educators are volunteers who, at best, receive an incentive in the form of lunch allowance, a bicycle or clothes. This is rarely sufficient to keep them interested for a longer period of time and leads to high turnover of peer educators, the need for repeated training of new volunteers and difficulties in finding sufficient volunteers. The discussion of monetary incentives is being held in most programmes using volunteers, with sustainability and unrealistic expectations about voluntarism being key concerns.

To sustain motivation, NGOs use a variety of learning methods and offer volunteers an added incentive by using different media, such as drama, songs, radio broadcasts, discussion fora and videos. Changing responsibilities of the volunteers on a regular basis also helps to build volunteer capacities and interest. Such responsibilities can include script writing, directing performances, performing, planning of outreach programmes, implementing radio broadcasts, carrying out research, and development of information, education and communication (IEC) materials. These experiences may also later facilitate the volunteers in finding employment.

Interest in becoming a volunteer increases with the possibility of learning from other volunteer groups through visits and workshops. Male and female peer educators consider this type of exposure very important, not only because they learn from each other, but also because it gives them opportunities to visit other places and acknowledges their status. Peer education is particularly attractive for girls because they develop new skills and receive new experiences, and it increases their self-esteem. An additional incentive is the recognition by adults that adolescents have a role to play in HIV/AIDS prevention, in some places leading to subsequent involvement of adolescents in community decision making.

Practice 19: HIV /AIDS awareness raising by youth group

The Sang Fan Wan Mai Youth Group started its peer education activities in 1996 as a result of a training programme that included the making and use of puppets for awareness raising activities. In the first few years, emphasis was put on developing stories for the puppet shows, training volunteers and doing performances. This focus changed to the use of different methods with different audiences including drama, story telling, radio broadcasts and sex education in schools. The volunteers do research to assess what issues are important in the target communities.and contact local expertise to participate when and where needed. New volunteers can choose to be trained in any type of activity. The result is a larger pool of volunteers, more volunteer groups and a large number of young people that have taken on a variety of responsibilities.

Monitoring of the impact of prevention activities needs more attention in programme development

Monitoring of the impact of awareness raising and prevention activities is an issue in all programmes in the toolkit. Most indicators are input indicators such as number of sessions or performances held, leaflets distributed, condoms distributed etc. These indicators do not measure impact and, consequently, there is no insight into whether a programme has reduced vulnerability to HIV in the target audience, the objective of most prevention programmes. Reasons why this is not being done include lack of funding and lack of technical expertise on how to carry out impact monitoring. Where impact is monitored, this is restricted to monitoring of some form of pre- and post-performance knowledge and attitudes, or to development of intervention plans, but rarely linked to the uptake of services.

Discussions with organizations contributing to the toolkit on the topic of monitoring indicated that from the start of prevention programmes, impact indicators and targets need to be developed, preferably with involvement of peer educators and staff. This also implies that a baseline assessment needs to be carried out. Actual monitoring should be done with the involvement of target audiences.

Home-based care

Local responses for care and support concentrate on the provision of home-based care. Home-based care is not a replacement of hospital care, but is part of a comprehensive continuum of prevention, care, treatment and support services that include the family, the community and various levels of health care providers. Because it is the first line of care, it is very important but, at the same time, most home-based care providers are volunteers and predominantly female. There are a number of issues in this type of care that are common to many of the programmes in the toolkit.

Home-based care increases access to care and support for HIV positive people and their families

With the increase of HIV and AIDS prevalence, the gap widens between demand for and availability of health care services. Many patients and family care-givers are too poor to access health care services. In response to this, health care service providers, community health workers or affected family members initiate home care programmes in which community volunteers are trained as care-givers. Many of the opportunistic infections that affect HIV positive people can be treated at home by trained volunteers who provide basic nursing care, as well as preventive therapies, guidance on nutritional requirements and palliative care. Home care volunteers give this care as part of more holistic support that includes social, psychological and counselling support not only for the patient but also for the family. This increases the quality of life of the HIV positive people, giving them dignity, respect and compassion. A specific category of home care volunteers are HIV positive people, this is discussed in the next section 'Involvement of HIV positive people increases effectiveness of prevention, care and impact mitigation activities'.

Where AIDS prevalence is high and home-based care has been established for a longer time period, volunteers more and more often become trainers of family care givers and focus on training, counselling and mentoring of these family members. Apart from training in care giving, the volunteers discuss basic facts about HIV/AIDS and prevention strategies. The increase of understanding within the families leads to a decrease in stigma and discrimination of the infected family member and a more caring household environment for the HIV positive person. Eventually, this also leads to a fertile environment for community development approaches that address stigma and discrimination and foster community commitment to address the prevention and impact of HIV/AIDS.

Care-givers are predominantly women and the extra burden of this care affects their own families' livelihood. The burden adversely affects women's physical and emotional health, while denying them opportunities to engage in economically productive work. The well being of other family members is undermined and tasks exacerbate poverty. In some programmes this has lead to the development of income-generating programmes specifically for care givers and more attention for psychological support for care volunteers.

Home-based care is most effective as part of a network of services

In order to provide the holistic support mentioned above, home-based care volunteers need to be able to link with public and private service providers: for health and nutritional aspects with health services; for counselling with health or social services; for spiritual guidance with faith-based organizations; for prevention with voluntary counselling and testing (VCT) services and schools; for income-generating activities with NGOs and community leaders; for orphan support with social services, faith-based organizations and community leaders; for legal support with specialized persons or agencies; and for training with specialized training institutions. The establishment of such networks requires effort, time and commitment. In many of the programmes included in the toolkit, these linkages do exist and they indicate that a clear understanding and agreement of the respective roles and responsibilities of the different organizations in the network is of crucial importance.

> **Practice 49: SEPO centre coordination of multi-sectoral AIDS prevention and care at district level, Zambia**
>
> In Zambia, in Livingstone district, an AIDS coordinating centre has been established as an initiative of the District Health Management Board. Through this centre responsibilities for training, support and supervision of home-based care volunteers are coordinated, provided by both mission-based health services and district health services. The centre also organizes peer education programmes, support groups of widows and orphans and HIV positive people, workplace education and counselling services. These different programmes link in with the VCT services that the centre provides for the whole district. The centre has been supporting income-generating activities for the home-based care volunteers, but these programmes have so far not been successful. Nutritional and material support for HIV positive people is channelled through the centre or through the mission, but made accessible for all home-based care groups..

Interest in volunteering increases with orientation and learning visits and specialized training

Mobilization of volunteers is an issue in all programmes. This is partly due to stigma, influenced by fear of transmission and lack of knowledge, and to lack of realization in the communities that much of the care for the sick can be effectively done at home. Actual mobilization is commonly done through community leadership, existing community groups or faith-based organizations and may take a long time. In Zambia, the Macha mission hospital now mobilizes volunteers in 'new' communities by taking leaders and interested community members to already established home-based care groups for orientation and this has led to an increased number of requests for training of home-based care volunteers from different communities (Practice 29).

Volunteers are usually selected on the basis of interest, residence in the community and ability to read and write. They receive an initial training (varying from three days to four weeks) covering HIV/AIDS basic knowledge, basic aspects of health care, opportunistic infections and their care requirements, basic counselling, nutrition and hygiene. Selected volunteers are given follow-up training covering specific aspects of care in more depth, such as DOTS treatment and counselling. Such specialized training, given by district health services or specialized NGOs, is highly valued by the volunteers because it is seen as a 'reward' for their activities and as a personal knowledge asset that is useful for the rest of their lives.

One aspect mentioned in all home care programmes in the toolkit is the provision of incentives for volunteers. This varies a lot and is often dependent on whether the home care initiative is taken by NGOs, the public health system or communities themselves. Incentives are given in the form of payments, bicycles, pens, books or materials for clothing, learning visits or loans for income-generating activities. There are two major issues to consider: sustainability and differentiation within a district. Where payment of financial incentives is provided through donor support, this may cease at the end of the project support unless the provision of incentives is taken over by the public health system.

When provision of incentives to volunteers differs within a district, it affects the interest and performance of those volunteers who receive less or no incentives. It is not realistic to expect home-based care volunteers, who are often very poor themselves, to continue providing care purely voluntarily when they realize others get paid and when they forfeit income-earning possibilities because of their volunteer work. Access to loans for income-generating activities can help in these cases, but this needs expert advice to and management skills of the volunteers.

Home-based care can only function as part of a continuum of care in which referral, supervision, training and supply of care kits are ensured

Volunteers are generally supervised by health staff during (bi)monthly visits in the community. The health staff visit patients that need special attention, giving on-the-job training to the volunteers. The visits are also used by the volunteers to organize discussions in the community on issues related to prevention, care and impact mitigation. The relationship with health staff is considered crucial by the volunteers because it gives them legitimacy in the eyes of the community and patients, and it strengthens their effectiveness as care givers because of the link with the health care system. The link to the health post and higher level health services is important because volunteers need to be ensured that adequate services are given to the patients. This is sometimes not the case because of lack of staff, lack of capacity, lack of drugs in the health facilities and a stigmatizing attitude of health workers towards AIDS patients.

Part of a good continuum of care is the provision of home care kits for the volunteers including drugs, gloves, soap, cotton gauze, and cleaning materials for the homes of patients. These basic home care kits are not always given and are frequently not being replenished when needed. This leads to frustration with the volunteers because the patients and their families have high expectations on the ability of the volunteers to provide care and alleviate suffering. Increased availability of funding at community level and above is needed to support a continuum of care that reaches out to people where they need it most: at home and in their communities.

Involvement of HIV positive people increases effectiveness of prevention, care and impact mitigation activities

Most HIV positive support groups involved in prevention and care activities in the toolkit have started at the instigation of a single individual that had the courage to disclose his or her status and which subsequently connected him/her to other infected people or their families (Ukraine: Practice 34; Thailand: Practice 35, 39, 45; Trinidad: Practice 47). Many of these initiators are women; men are less likely to become involved in care activities. Initially activities focus on care giving, especially in situations where home-based care is non existent as in Ukraine, and on the provision of mutual psycho-social support either in group sessions or during home visits. Some groups are supported by outside counsellors, but in most programmes HIV positive members themselves receive training in medical care and/or counselling in order to provide care and support. This is most effective when there are links with other

local responses to hiv/aids from a gender perspective

sectors such as traditional healers, village health volunteers, health workers, schools and faith-based organizations that each give a different kind of support.

Counselling by HIV positive people is crucial in restoring hope and empowering infected persons to fight for their life and to give meaning to the rest of their lives. The mutual support in these groups helps people to disclose their HIV-status to their families and not to bear the burden of their infection alone. Counselling is also provided to help families to accept the situation and to link them with various support services.

In Thailand and Brazil groups have started very effective income-generating projects and saving and loan schemes, also benefiting other vulnerable groups and involving the community at large (Practice 39, 40, 45). These efforts help to create understanding and compassion and mobilize community support for HIV positive people. It has to be stressed, however, that in all programmes outside support from donors and/or NGOs has been instrumental in getting these activities organized.

Practice 45: Support from monks to a Positive Women's Group, Thailand

The abbot in a village in northern Thailand assisted the 35 members of the Positive Women's Group by funding their attendance in a government vocational training on tailoring and handicraft. After the training, a workshop was constructed on the temple grounds through donations of the community, the temple and the district administration. Later, sewing machines and spinning wheels were bought with donations and group income from product sales. Sales were limited, but a visit of a Japanese monk to the abbot resulted in a 10 year order for material and ready-made kimonos from Japan. Training for production of material and kimonos was given by a Japanese consultant. At present, there is so much work that also other community members, especially poor groups such as widows and the elderly, are involved in the work and all earn an income from the outputs produced.

Almost all HIV positive support groups are involved in prevention activities in their communities. Through presentation in the community in schools, churches, temples and at community gatherings, HIV positive people (men and women, although the latter are more numerous) are actively involved in increasing community understanding on HIV/AIDS. Everywhere the impact of such public talks is tremendous and is reported to help decrease stigma and discrimination in the communities.

HIV positive people in one group in Thailand have been trained by an NGO to counsel and support HIV positive people that are receiving ART (Practice 35). Doctors in the hospital give a monthly check-up and prescription, while support is organized by the trained HIV positive men and women in the form of counselling, advice on treatment of side effects and simple opportunistic infections, as well as monitoring of adherence. They have become so experienced that they frequently have arguments on regimens prescribed by the (less experienced) doctors. The empowerment and the ability to deal effectively with their own condition makes a difference in the mental and physical state of these HIV positive people. Other support focuses on the use of traditional herbs, certain types of food and physical exercises to remain healthy.

Faith-based organizations have a crucial role in instigating and supporting local responses to HIV/AIDS

In most countries covered in the toolkit, faith-based organizations form the spiritual and social backbone of society and are well placed to respond to the epidemic. Many of these organizations are involved in HIV/AIDS prevention, care and support programmes. They influence the attitude of community members towards HIV positive people and the extent to which communities regard HIV/AIDS as a community concern rather than an individual or family concern: their spiritual leadership can be the motor for positive community responses or the source of stigma and discrimination. Key aspects relate to the inclusion of prevention activities and to training of staff of faith-based organizations.

Faith-based organizations incorporate prevention in their care and support programmes

Religious organizations that promote a positive response are incorporating HIV/AIDS care and support in the principles of their faith. They guide their members to show compassion and to support those infected and affected in their communities. Initially faith-based organizations concentrated on spiritual support and health care to HIV positive people. There are now practices from Thailand and Zambia on home-based care programmes supported from the temple and the church (Practice 1, 45, 29, 30). Where faith-based organizations manage hospitals and health care facilities, as is the case in Zambia and Uganda, these mission hospitals were among the first to establish home-based care teams reaching out to remote parts of the districts and establishing a well-functioning continuum of care.

Faith-based organizations that have been involved over a longer period in this type of care, are seen to change their focus to a more comprehensive approach in which prevention and community development in the community as a whole, is added to spiritual support and health care for HIV positive people and their families. Home-based care volunteers and community outreach workers from faith-based organizations are addressing prevention with a focus on HIV/AIDS awareness raising, on different methods for prevention and on traditional cultural practices that increase susceptibility for HIV infection, such as sexual cleansing. In line with the doctrines of their faith and the official positions of the religious hierarchies, the organizations emphasize abstinence and being faithful as the preferred strategies for HIV prevention. But many of the organizations documented in the toolkit also provide information on condom use and on places where condoms are available for free or for sale. The basis of their prevention activities is to provide information to people to make their own informed choices. Included in a prevention strategy is also promotion of VCT and information on the advantages of knowing one's status. This has led to an increase in uptake of VCT, supported by a decrease in stigma in the communities as a result of the care and prevention strategies that led the communities to address HIV/AIDS as a collective issue that affects them all.

local responses to hiv/aids from a gender perspective

Training is required for staff of faith-based organizations to expand their traditional role to become facilitators of community AIDS competence

The faith-based organizations are training their male and female staff in workshops to take on their additional roles as facilitators and to become promoters of a multi-sectoral approach that involves government, religious organizations, NGOs and the community to address impacts and develop effective approaches for prevention. In Thailand, the Sangha Metta project was initiated by monks in 1997 in response to the need for monks to have a more active role in HIV/AIDS prevention and care. Taking the Buddhist teachings as their inspiration, they concluded that a core aspect of HIV/AIDS was ignorance about the condition both among those infected and the general public. In line with their traditional role as teachers, they decided they could teach both groups about its realities.

> **Practice 1: Buddhist approach to prevention and care**
> In the Sangha Metta project, training seminars are conducted with monks, nuns and novices. Topics covered are basic knowledge on HIV/AIDS, the impact on the community and development and its socioeconomic impacts. This is then applied to Buddhist teachings to increase understanding. Monks and lay people engaged in community development work are invited to talk and also this is applied to Buddhist teachings. HIV positive people are invited to talk about their experiences, their needs and wants from the monks and the community. The training also covers participatory skills, life skills education and social management skills. In contrast with their traditional formal roles (where the monks wait for the community to come to them), the project trains monks to have a more active role in community work. Using Buddhist ethics as their guideline, they now teach villagers how to avoid high-risk behaviour, help to set up support groups, train people with HIV/AIDS in handicrafts, donate their alms and take care of AIDS orphans. Because local people are accustomed to telling monks their troubles, many HIV positive people who have not disclosed, come to them for advice and can be referred to support groups and public assistance programmes. 'HIV-friendly' temples encourage HIV positive people to participate in community activities. This more active role among monks is strengthening trust between them and the people, and leads to greater grass roots participation in solving problems at the local level.

In Zambia, the Christian Health Association of Zambia (CHAZ) is conducting training sessions where male and female staff from missions across the country, involved in HIV/AIDS activities, come together to share their experiences and learn from each other. Participatory approaches are taught for use in the community as well as strategies to develop networks of stakeholders in HIV/AIDS that take the needs of HIV positive people as the starting point.

Sharing of knowledge and learning increases scaling up of effective approaches of local responses to HIV/AIDS

The use of participatory approaches increases learning from within and leads to commitment and ownership of interventions by the communities

In the response to HIV/AIDS, participatory techniques are particularly effective in addressing issues that need reflection and action by communities, while they build on local knowledge and experience. The techniques are always gender sensitive, because women and men, often in different age groups, work on their own assessment of an dentified problem and are then guided to present their results to the group at large. This ensures that the views of these different groups are expressed and form the basis of community strategies. The techniques are found to increase understanding of the vulnerability of different groups in the community and this in turn leads to increased commitment and ownership of interventions by communities and/or specific groups. The techniques are helpful in assisting the community to understand the underlying causes of an identified problem and the barriers that exist for different groups to solutions of that problem.

Technique 1: AIDS trend appraisal

The technique 'AIDS trend appraisal' helps communities to assess changes in relation to different aspects of HIV/AIDS in the community (such as knowledge about HIV/AIDS, stigma, number of orphans, condom use, onset of sexual activity) over time, marking 5 years ago, the present and in 5 years time). It facilitates identification of interrelationships between these aspects and between other issues in the community (poverty, lack of employment, lack of access to basic services) and gives insight in the difference in perceptions among various groups in the community (men, women, youth). The technique helps to raise awareness on the impact of HIV/AIDS at community level, and helps to mobilize and plan for interventions at this level.

During the country visits to organizations, it became clear that NGOs, which are already using participatory techniques and have experienced and confident facilitators, are very eager to try out new and different techniques. Facilitators who have only been trained once in participatory techniques (and this is often the case in small NGOs) tend to apply the methodology as 'rote' facilitation where the session itself becomes the output and not the planned activities that are the result of the session. For organizations that have not been trained at all and for those that have only been trained once, it is therefore advisable to plan for training and retraining in sessions where the participants can also learn from each other's experiences in using the techniques.

Strategies need to be developed for structured sharing and learning

All organizations contributing to the toolkit have stressed the importance of strategies to share knowledge and learn from each other within and between countries. This does not happen automatically and can only be effectively done if it is well planned and funds are available for this purpose. In most countries, in the capital cities or other large cities, organizations involved in HIV/AIDS are aware of each other's programmes and activities, even when these are carried out in rural areas. But in the rural areas, many organizations work in relative isolation unless networks have been established. Usually such networks exist because there is an umbrella organization that functions as a secretariat for member organizations (such as CHAZ in Zambia), or network organizations have been specifically established with the aim to share and create knowledge and build capacity. This is the case with the Uganda Network of AIDS Service Organizations (UNASO), the project Somos of Grupo Dignidade in Brazil and AIDSnet in Thailand. Also in Trinidad such a network is in the process of being established.

It is very important to ensure that knowledge sharing and dissemination is not restricted to the national level, although national level agencies have their own role in this: the development of strategies to facilitate local responses, learning and mainstreaming, coordination, advocacy. District level agencies have a different role: translation of national and international policies into district level policies/practices, feedback on good experiences into national policy level, training, advocacy and facilitation. But for local responses, the focus has to be on decentralized levels that are directly working with local communities that are faced with HIV/AIDS. Local initiatives are also the source of knowledge creation as this is the level where different approaches are being tried out. How this is best done depends on the situation in the country. A main barrier to knowledge sharing and mutual assistance, however, is competition over scarce resources. Specifically at community and sub-district level, organizations are competing for donor funds. One way this can be addressed is to prioritize those projects for funding in which more than one NGO is involved, as is being proposed in Soroti District, Uganda.

Strategies that have proven to work in the countries visited, include structured study visits, organizational mentoring, apprenticeships, training workshops on specific themes, thematic networks, dissemination of good practices through newsletters and facilitation teams. Such facilitation teams, for instance in Zambia, consist of a rotating group of people active in the field of HIV/AIDS that respond to invitation from districts, communities or organizations. They facilitate stakeholders coming together and developing strategies that involve different organizations and provide links to organizations that can help on specific issues. Moreover, they share responses that have been developed in other parts of the country. However, it has proven to be difficult to find funding for this kind of initiative.

Conclusions

While it has for a long time been assumed that people and communities would respond effectively to HIV/AIDS if they have access to adequate information and support, we have now learned that there are a number of key factors that are required for an effective and sustained local response.

Men and women in the communities need to feel ownership of the problem that they are facing with respect to HIV/AIDS and of the interventions that they plan to address the problem. Participatory techniques are helpful in guiding men and women to analyse their own situation and to establish their needs and priorities, in order to plan interventions. The use of these techniques also facilitates understanding of how men and women are affected differently by the epidemic, not only in their vulnerabilities but also in impact. For example, women face more barriers to protect themselves as a consequence of the unequal power structure within relationships; women are more likely to face stigma and discrimination within the household and within the community; women are predominantly involved in care for AIDS patients and orphans. Women may need specific support to overcome traditional inhibitions to speak out in public and to overcome male dominance. Successful use of the techniques requires facilitation by a person or an organization from within or outside the community. Such people may include NGO staff, district staff or people from faith-based or community-based organizations and they should be men and women. All facilitators need to be well trained and this cannot be done during a single training. This also requires follow-up and refresher training.

There is a limit to what people and communities can do on their own. For local responses to be effective, there is a need for local partnerships and interaction between communities and service providers. Raising awareness through peer education programmes is a first step on the road to behaviour change. Other factors that need to be addressed in a gender-sensitive manner are increased access to services such as STI clinics, sex education and life skills education in schools, opportunities for income generation, and involvement in community decision making. Home-based care by community volunteers hinges on an effective and dependable continuum of care in which health care facilities at different levels are involved, but also has to address the negative impact voluntarism has on care-givers and their families. The division of responsibilities and tasks at different levels has to be clear and agreed upon. In addition, care and support to HIV positive people and their families has to respond to their needs and this implies holistic support, including social, psychological and counselling support, the creation of a supportive community environment and access to basic services. Service providers thus need to assess how their services can mitigate the impact of HIV/AIDS and respond to emerging needs in the communities.

HIV positive people, men and women, have a very important role to play not only in awareness raising and prevention activities, but also in planning and implementation of care and support activities. Most HIV positive organizations have been started by very courageous individuals, but as a group they are more likely to be able to reduce stigma and discrimination in their communities. They need support from faith-based organizations and their spiritual guidance is often crucial in mobilizing communities.

A supportive environment for local responses includes political and spiritual leadership, mass communication and the adoption and implementation of supportive legislation, especially addressing the protection of women and children. However, above all, it needs scaling up of locally available services and financial resources. It is completely unrealistic to expect communities that are already stretched to the limit of their capacity, to be able to address the impact of HIV/AIDS without financial support from outside. Too many programmes are dependent on volunteer support and it is clear that it becomes more and more difficult to find such volunteers, especially in the hardest hit countries. It is also not realistic to expect that people who are poor and have difficulties in providing a living for their families, can spend so much of their time and energy in taking care of HIV positive people and their families. It needs concerted effort to direct financial and other resources to the local communities that need this support most.

Finally, strategies for knowledge sharing, learning and knowledge creation need to be developed and supported in order for organizations and communities to adapt and apply interventions that have proven to be effective. The practices and techniques in the toolkit will help in this process. There are numerous approaches for knowledge sharing as mentioned in the section 'Sharing of knowledge and learning increases scaling up of effective approaches of local responses to HIV/AIDS but they have to be planned and implemented in a structured way with good facilitation and funds to support organizations to take part in this process.

References

Wegelin-Schuringa, M. and G. Tiendrebeogo (eds), 'Techniques and practices for local responses to HIV/AIDS: UNAIDS toolkit. 2 parts. Amsterdam/Geneva, KIT/UNAIDS, 2004. http://www.kit.nl/publishers/html/publications_online.asp

Overview of practices for local responses to HIV/AIDS

No	Practice	Key words
Prevention		
1	Buddhist approach to prevention and care	Faith-based organizations, community, training, prevention, care, Thailand
2	Club Cool	Youth, sexual and reproductive health, income-generating activities, Haiti
3	Community Art vs. AIDS	Youth, community, contest, prevention, care and support, arts, Togo
4	Community Centre for IDUs	Intravenous drug users (IDUs), prevention, syringe exchange, counselling, Ukraine
5	Condom 'Krew'	Youth, sexual and reproductive health, condom promotion, carnival, Trinidad
6	Cross Border project	Truck drivers, prevention, condom promotion, Hong Kong
7	'The Living Room'	Youth friendly clinic, sexual and reproductive health, Trinidad
8	Drop-in centre for sex workers	Commercial sex workers, prevention, skills training, social and legal protection, Thailand
9	Each one, teach one	Men having sex with men (MSM), prevention, safer sex practices, Hong Kong
10	'Jus Once' an interactive HIV/AIDS awareness production	Community, prevention, myths, sexuality, drama and arts, Trinidad
11	Life skills education in a poor suburb in São Paulo	Prevention, life skills education, teacher training, Brazil
12	Meakaotom Youth Group	Youth, peer education, prevention, Thailand
13	Migrant workers prevention and care	Migrant workers, prevention, care, Brazil
14	Mobile VCT clinic	Voluntary counselling and testing (VCT), prevention, India
15	Prison setting prevention and care	Prison, care, prevention, Zambia
16	HIV/AIDS protection of young male prostitutes	Street boys, prevention, Brazil
17	Rap against silence	Youth, prevention, music contest, radio, arts, Togo
18	Resource centre for youth	Youth, peer education, prevention, Uganda
19	Sang Phan Wan Mai Youth Group	Youth, prevention, peer education, puppet shows, radio, schools, Thailand
20	Sex industry outreach	Sex workers, clients, sex industry, prevention, Hong Kong
21	Toco Youth Sexuality Project	Youth, community, prevention, peer education, Trinidad
22	VCT at MSM saunas	MSM, VCT, Hong Kong
23	Voucher scheme	MSM, IDUs, sex workers, sexual and reproductive health, access to services, Nicaragua
24	Wear to care	Youth, schools, prevention, social mobilization, arts, Togo
25	Young people's movement	Youth, peer education, prevention, Nepal
26	Youth learning to take care in a poor neighbourhood in São Paulo	Youth, prevention, peer education, Brazil
27	Video Documentary of HIV/AIDS Projects, 'Choice or Chance'	Youth organizations, documentation, Trinidad

local responses to hiv/aids from a gender perspective

Care and treatment

28	Group Therapy, 'Show you care, Take care of yourself and others'	People Living With HIV/AIDS (PLWH), group therapy, care and support, Trinidad
29	Macha mission home-based care and prevention	Home-based care, prevention, Zambia
30	Maramba home-based care and prevention	Home-based care, prevention, Zambia
31	Masaka ARV provision	ART, Uganda
32	Mpigi home-based care	Home-based care, Uganda
33	Nursery for orphans and children affected by AIDS	Orphans, faith-based organizations, care and support, ART, Trinidad
34	Psycho-social and home care for PLWH	PLWH, home-based care, psycho-social support, Ukraine
35	Sai Samphan management of ART by PLWH group	PLWH, counselling, ART, Thailand

Support and mitigation

36	Access integrated child support Thailand	Children, orphans, care takers, counselling, treatment, support,
37	Balcão de direitos (Rights Corner)	Legal advice, law, human rights, partnerships, Brazil
38	'Child is Life' Project	PLWH, adolescents, orphans and vulnerable children, psychosocial support, skills training, Brazil
39	PLWH Health and Income generating activities	PLWH, community, income-generating activities, Thailand
40	Co-operative of PLWH for producing school uniforms	PLWH, municipality, income-generating activities, Brazil
41	Farm school for orphans	Orphans, education, start-up assistance, income generating activities, Uganda
42	Counselling and skills training in Karaope House	PLWH, counselling, skills training, Zambia
43	Support to orphan girls in Kara Umoyo	Orphans, counselling, skills training, employment, Zambia
44	Orphan feeding scheme	Orphans and vulnerable children, nutrition, psycho-social support, South Africa
45	Support from monks to HIV positive women groupThailand	Faith-based organizations, PLWH, income-generating activities, Partnerships and coordination
46	NGO and Local Government cooperation	District, multi-sectoral cooperation, Uganda
47	People Living with HIV/AIDS Coming Together in the Caribbean	PLWH, networking, leadership, Trinidad, Caribbean
48	Networking and training of MSM NGOs: Projeto Somos	MSM, community, mobilization, training, scaling-up, Brazil
49	SEPO Centre, district coordination	District, coordination, prevention, care, Zambia
50	Soroti Network of AIDS Service Organizations (SONASO)	NGO network, advocacy, district, coordination, Uganda

Source: Wegelin-Schuringa, M. and G. Tiendrebeogo, 'Techniques and practices for local responses to HIV/AIDS: UNAIDS toolkit'. Amsterdam, KIT Publishers, 2004. www.kit.nl/publishers/html/publications_online.asp

6 Stigma, discrimination and violence amongst female sex workers and men who have sex with men in Andhra Pradesh, India

There is no support available to fight against discrimination and violence. How can we go and tell people that we are prostitutes and these are the problems we are facing and so help us? They do not help us even if we say we are doing this work as there is no other way for us. In case we face any problems then we suppress it within ourselves but we don't go to anyone for help... Now I am telling you about my situation, will you provide me with a livelihood so that I can get relieved of all these harassments? You will only take this information and give it to your office. There is no one to help me out. Even if I go along with political parties they don't help me.
(Testimony of a female sex worker)

One-third of people living with the human immune deficiency virus (HIV) are in countries that do not yet have generalized epidemics. Even a small increase in infection rates in countries without generalized epidemics, especially populous ones, would represent a dramatic worsening of the global burden of the acquired immune deficiency syndrome (AIDS). Thus, there is an urgent need to reduce HIV infections in relatively low-prevalence countries that are put at risk by the growing HIV pandemic (Ainsworth and Over 1999).

In the late 1990s, there were an estimated 4 million HIV-infected individuals in India. By the end of 2003, this had risen to an estimated 5.1 million, the second highest number outside South Africa (UNAIDS 2004; NACO 2004). Most (80%) infections in India are attributed to heterosexual transmission. HIV surveillance data indicate that the prevalence of HIV among antenatal clinic attendants is approximately 2% in Andhra Pradesh. Among attendees of clinics for sexually transmitted infections (STIs), HIV rates of 20-40% have been reported in several areas.

Female sex workers and men who have sex with men

Female sex workers and men who have sex with men have been identified as two key populations that India cannot ignore in its effort to prevent the spread of the HIV epidemic. About 1.1% of the women in the adult population in India could be engaged in sex work (NACO 2003) and homosexual behaviour in the general population is estimated to range between 4-11% (Verma and Collumbien 2004). While by all anecdotal evidence stigma constitutes an important barrier to efforts to mobilize and empower these populations in order to prevent the spread of HIV, there exists very little empirical evidence on the nature, antecedents and the extent of stigma. Most imperfectly understood is the programmatic response that will be needed to reduce stigma.

stigma, discrimination and violence

In order to contextualize this study, it is necessary to provide a brief background on the categories of men who have sex with men in India. Unlike the western gay community, the homosexual scene in India is diverse in nature (Asthana and Oostvogels 2001). There are specific and exclusive 'sexual identities' in opposition to heterosexuality, known by various names depending upon regional background and sexual preferences. While there is a distinct category of men who have sex with men who identify themselves as 'gay', they are generally English speaking from middle to upper class socioeconomic backgrounds. According to Shivananda Khan, most same sex relationships between men in South Asia are based on gendered self-identities and sex roles. The most visible of these same sex identities involves men who identify themselves as *kothis* (Khan 2005). *Kothis* are considered to be the receptive partners in same sex interactions. It is postulated that most *kothis*, if not all, are engaged in sex work, come largely from low-income groups and cut across caste, religion and region (UNESCO 2001). Some of the *kothis* are also known to have fixed *babus* or partners. This paper deals with this sub-section of men who have sex with men, i.e. *kothis*, who are explicitly feminized. *Kothis* are found in large numbers in the project areas and the project itself is focusing on them.

Stigma and discrimination: barriers to prevention

It is increasingly recognized that HIV and AIDS-related stigma and discrimination pose one of the greatest challenges to effective prevention and treatment (UNAIDS 2001; Parker and Aggleton 2003). Stigma and discrimination are rooted in shame and fear. Shame because of the taboos surrounding the modes of transmission, namely sex and injecting drug use, and fear because the disease is known to be deadly, and because of lack of knowledge about the disease (Piot 2001). One of the major sources of stigma comes from the moral judgement about sexual behaviour that is responsible for the infection. Female sex workers and men who have sex with men also face severe forms of stigma because they are commonly labelled as the carrier of the virus. Stigma builds upon and reinforces existing inequalities within societies resulting in social exclusion, further marginalizing vulnerable groups. For the purpose of this paper, the forms and consequences of stigma can be equated with discrimination or enacted stigma.

There exists a large and growing body of literature that seeks to define and analyse the nature of stigma, not only in relation to HIV but also in relation to other stigmatized conditions such as leprosy, epilepsy and tuberculosis (TB) (KIT 2004). A landmark study dating back to the early 1960s points out the role of stigma in societies to confirm the 'normalcy' of the majority through the devaluation of the 'other' (Goffman 1963). Goffman goes on to describe three types of stigma:
- 'abominations of the body', or stigma related to physical deformities;
- stigma related to 'blemishes of individual character', such as people who are considered to be weak-willed, to have unnatural passions, or to be dishonest; and
- 'tribal stigma', or stigma relating to race, nation or religion, or membership of a despised social group.

In a more recent study, Parker and Aggleton (2003), describe how stigma can be used by dominant groups to legitimize and perpetuate inequalities, such as those based on gender, age, sexual orientation, class, race or ethnicity. In this case, stigma is seen as a framework through which relations of power and control are produced and reproduced.

Compound stigma (also referred to as multiple stigma) is HIV stigma that is layered on top of pre-existing stigmas, frequently toward homosexuals, sex workers, injecting drug users, women, and youth (Herek and Capitanio 1997; Herek et al 2002; Boer and Emons 2004; Brown et al 2004; Kalichman and Simbayi 2004; Nyblade 2004). Enacted stigma has been defined by some as discrimination; discrimination is not separate from stigma but the end result of the process of stigma, or '... the negative acts that result from stigma that serve to devalue and reduce the life chance of the stigmatized' (USAID 2005).

A recent study in four countries, Zambia, Ethiopia, Tanzania and Vietnam, exploring HIV and AIDS-related stigma found that:

> Looking across contexts, are commonalities in what causes stigma, the forms in which stigma is expressed and the consequences of stigma...Variations that stem from differences in language, culture and epidemic history are largely of nuance and degree rather than substance. (Ogden and Nyblade 2005)

Consequences of stigma for individuals living with HIV/AIDS, their families, treatment and prevention efforts are also similar across countries. Loss of livelihood, for instance, for individuals and their families is a recurring theme, as is loss of reputation, internalized stigma, loss of options around marriage and child bearing, and the role that stigma plays as an obstacle for getting tested for HIV or for disclosure to others.

In summary, stigma can be understood from a variety of perspectives and can be seen as enacted, perceived and self-internalized. As it is multidimensional in nature, has deep rooted causes and represents a vicious cycle of increasing stigmatization, it must be tackled in a holistic and multidisciplinary fashion.

The study

The data for the present paper are drawn from a nested study within a larger Frontiers Prevention Project (FPP) research project in Andhra Pradesh, India. The FPP is based on the principle of providing a comprehensive package of interventions in geographically defined sites that are focused on population groups that are key to the dynamics of the HIV epidemic. These include female sex workers, men who have sex with men, and people living with HIV/AIDS. These populations, or key populations, are key not only in the sense that they are more vulnerable to infection and onward transmission, but also because without their mobilization and empowerment, the epidemic will continue to grow (Global HIV Prevention Working Group 2003; Campbell and Mzaidume 2001). Fundamental to the entire approach proposed by the FPP is the principle that programmes and services will be more effective when implemented in the context of meaningful community participation, mobilization and involvement at all levels.

This paper describes the nature, antecedents and the extent of stigma and discrimination among female sex workers and a cultural category of men who have sex with men. We have presented the findings of these two populations together because both involve strong gender dimension of stigma and discrimination; both deal in a trade that is illegal; and both are highly stigmatized and therefore hidden. The category of men considered here identify themselves as *kothis* or 'not men', namely men who are sexually penetrated by their male partners who are referred to as *panthis* or 'real men'.

Methodology

The data for the study was collected through in-depth interviews and focus group discussions with female sex workers and *kothis*, selected from eight intervention sites of FPP located in eight districts of Andhra Pradesh. In each site, 4 interviews were carried out with each respondent type, making a total of 32 interviews with sex workers and 32 with *kothis*. Before beginning each interview, the aim of the study was explained to participants; they then signed an informed consent form, agreeing to participate. In addition, two focus group discussions for female sex workers and two for *kothis* were conducted in each of the eight sites.

Descriptive data was analysed using an analytical framework that delineated the following themes: social capital; self-esteem; stigma, discrimination and violence; knowledge, attitude and practice regarding HIV prevention; and awareness and utilization of services. Each theme was defined in operational terms and two independent coders coded the transcripts using Atlas ti software. Verbatim quotes from the respondents were used extensively to substantiate a particular interpretation and to arrive at a high level of inter-coder consensus. Themes, sub-themes and verbatim quotes therefore constitute the basic data sheet for drawing interpretations for the present analysis.

The majority of female sex workers taking part in the study was illiterate (21 out of 32, married or separated/widowed (23 out of 32) and belonged to age range 18-40 years. The majority of *kothis* interviewed was literate (18 out of 32); half of them were married (16 out of 32) and belonged to the 18-52 year age group. Most men engaged in multiple partner sex that involved cruising in well-defined sites. However, many of these encounters were reportedly non-commercial in nature as opposed to the female sex workers where sex was primarily commercial.

Language, expressions and forms of stigma, discrimination and violence

There are a variety of terms in local languages that are used to stigmatize female sex workers and *kothis*. Some of the terms that were identified during the in-depth interviews for female sex workers include *paitalu, lanja, chedindi, thirugumothulu* and *lanjalu*. These are extremely demeaning terminologies to imply that a woman who engages in sex work is highly demoralized and morally corrupt. The stigmatizing terms used for female sex workers have strong moral underpinning and arise from the construct of a femininity that is expected to remain devoted to one man and one family. Within this construct of gender and sexuality, men can have many female sexual partners and can still be viewed as a masculine man, while multiple sexual relations for women does not form part of the femininity construct.

Terms used for *kothis*, on the other hand, include *gandugadu, fifty-fifty, chaakka*, and *kojja* among many others. Interestingly, demeaning terms used to stigmatize *kothis* do not carry heavy moral implications. Rather, they tend to condemn a man who behaves like a woman in sexual relations by receiving penetrative sex. It is evident that it is the 'feminization' of a man that is less socially acceptable than the sexual behaviour *per se*. Indian literature on homosexuality suggests that men who penetrate other men are described with much greater respect *(panthi)* than those who are penetrated *(kothi)*, creating some kind of hierarchy on the lines of gender among homosexuals.

Most respondents were subjected to various forms of stigmatizing comments or gestures in their everyday life. Of these, degrading comments which are perceived as bringing shame or loss of honour, labelling or addressing the respondents by demeaning terms ridiculing or making fun of their identity and criticism are more commonly reported. Other forms reported include: sarcastic comments, teasing, hatred and contemptuous looks.

Both female sex workers and *kothis* very commonly reported public expressions of stigmatizing language. Female sex workers are also stigmatized for belonging to a particular caste, which is labelled for accepting and encouraging female sex work, the *Bhogam* and *Dommara* castes. Some of the respondents reported that although they do not belong to a particular caste, they are often referred to by the name of the caste in order to imply that they deserve to be sex workers.

Both the groups reported having experienced avoidance and isolation, expulsion from rented homes, denial of services, opportunities and support. Avoidance and isolation are the most common forms of discriminatory behaviour reported by both sex workers and *kothis*: refusing to speak with the respondent; severing existing ties once their identity is revealed; not inviting respondents to social functions or attending functions organized by the respondents; not touching objects used by respondent; and not allowing respondents entry to their houses and not entering houses of the respondents. As female sex workers revealed:

> *People degrade us. They criticize us saying that we are the ones with loose morals and would sleep with anyone for money. They think that we have bad characters.*

> *People think that we do not have any values. They say that we indulge in drinking and sex work. They do not talk to us and also do not allow us to live in the streets where they reside.*

> *Every person has something to say about us. They say that we take ten people along with us when we die, that their children would get spoiled because of us.*

An overwhelming majority of respondents from both the groups reported that they have experienced violence from various sources, including from the police. Common forms of violent behaviour experienced include: beating, verbal abuse and threats;

stigma, discrimination and violence

theft of money and valuables; rape, 'unnatural sex' by force, coercive sex with multiple persons, and coercive sex without condoms; and electric shocks to the body, hitting with stones and other objects etc.

Sources of stigma, discrimination and violence

Perpetuators of stigma as reported by the respondents include: family members, spouses/partners, friends, health care personnel, government officials, house owners, colleagues, police and rowdies (noisy troublemakers). There are subtle differences in the experience of stigma between female sex workers and *kothis*. The form and severity of stigmatizing behaviour also varies depending on the perpetuators of stigma. While the general public, neighbours, family members, relatives and health care personnel are reported as the major source of stigma and discrimination; clients, police and rowdies are more commonly implicated in the more extreme forms of violence experienced by the respondents. We will briefly describe some of the important sources of stigma, discrimination and violence as they relate to female sex-workers and *kothis* in our study population.

Spouses/partners, family members, peers, friends and clients

A significant number of the female sex workers were currently married, separated or widowed. Some were engaged in sex work with the knowledge of their husbands. Some of the currently unmarried respondents had a regular partner. In local parlance, they are known as temporary husbands. These temporary husbands are normally aware of the respondent's occupation and, in many cases, work as a gatekeeper to broker clients. Lack of help from the husband to support the family, abandonment by husbands, alcoholism and abuse by husbands were often cited as reasons for taking up sex work. In some cases, husbands deserted their wives once they came to know that the latter was engaged in sex work. Respondents reported that they experienced degrading comments about their choice of work, physical abuse by husbands/ partners, and coercion by husbands/partners to part with the earnings, and forceful abortion when the husband suspects that the child is not his. As one literate sex worker testifies:

> *My husband married twice. My husband is an alcoholic and doesn't take care of the house. He lives with the other woman. He beats me also. I am not educated I can't get a job and to feed my daughter I am doing this work.*

Many of the *kothis* were married with children. While some wives are aware that their husbands have sex with other men, most do not know. Often, their wives deserted them when their sexuality was revealed. Married or not, many of the men had regular partners, sometime more than one. As *kothis* bear witness:

> Kothis *face torture from their partners. The partner insists that the he should not go to any other person (for sex) and has to stay only with him.*

> *When my partner beats me I feel helpless. I have to keep silent, as he is stout to beat him back.*

Female sex workers experienced more stigma from family members and relatives than *kothis*. It is however interesting that a much higher proportion of female sex workers in our study had reportedly revealed to their family members that they are engaged in sex work. While this disclosure had helped them to cope with their work situation, it had also led to violence from within the family.

Among families of the *kothis*, there is generally an acceptance of their sexual identity. Compared to female sex workers, fewer *kothis* who are sex workers revealed the nature of their occupation to their families. Stigma and discrimination experienced by female sex workers from family and relatives include: derogatory comments, criticism and ridicule from spouses, parents or in-laws; abandonment by husbands and their families; expulsion from parental and marital homes; parents and in-laws not visiting them and they not being allowed in the homes of the former; not being invited to family functions and family members keeping away from functions organized by the respondents; refusal to provide any help or support in times of need etc. Stigma and discrimination experienced by *kothis* from family and relatives include: degrading comments and ridicule pertaining to sexuality of the respondent, avoidance and isolation at social functions, denial of support, and desertion by wives.

Female sex workers were found to have a very limited number of friends. Of those who did, they were females and often peers, and were usually reported as persons in whom the respondent could trust and confide. On the other hand, many *kothis* reported that their friends were a source of stigma and discrimination; they ridiculed and teased them because of their feminine characteristics. Some reported that their friends felt uncomfortable with them and did not want to be seen with them in public. Others reported that their friends severed all ties with them and isolated them once their identity became known:

> *All my close school friends who were always there with me stopped talking to me after they came to know that I am a* [kothi].

> *Usually my friends discriminate me. They are disgusted that I am doing this and left me. No matter how much I help them, it always happens.*

Peers also tend to stigmatize and discriminate amongst themselves; this behaviour is essentially based on difference. Amongst *kothis*, differences are based on social status, age groups and physical looks. Generally *kothis* engaged in commercial sex work are looked down upon. Despite active involvement in peer groups (see below), most *kothis* have little or no trust in their peers. Some of the reasons expressed include: frequent change in partners, jealousy, fear that other peers may entice his partner, lack of support and fear of their secrets being revealed. As a result, peer groups are unstable and members move from one group to the other. Differences among female sex workers exist on basis of earning potential, caste, whether they are locals or outsiders and between home and street-based sex workers. As in the case of *kothis*, there is very little trust among peers. Experiences of being cheated, backbiting, feelings of jealousy, bad character, competition for customers, lack of support were some of the reasons cited by the female sex workers for mistrust in peers.

An overwhelming majority of the respondents in both groups reported that they were stigmatized and subjected to violence by clients. Some sex workers reported that clients who had sex with them previously would abuse them in public and reveal their identity to others. Most of them reported varying degrees of violence at the hands of clients. They were beaten up, forced to have sex with multiple clients, robbed of their money and valuables, raped, coerced to have sex without condom or payment, forced to have unnatural sex, abused and harassed by clients. Some of the men reported that clients sometime threatened to reveal the respondents identity to their family and blackmailed them. Both women and *kothis* report similar experiences:

> Clients hit [kothis] *saying that we should do well as we are taking money. They pull our hair. Some times they don't give money. They say that they don't want to use condoms. They keep asking us to do as they want, offering us more money.*

> Clients who are in drunken state hit us a lot. We [female sex workers] go with clients to some remote places to have sex. They're taking the advantage of deserted area. Clients rob our money and go away.

That the sex workers and *kothis* are constantly living under a threat of violence from clients is readily acknowledged by NGO staff and other gatekeepers:

> People come to them and have sex. Sometimes some of them batter the sex workers and take away their money. Sometimes clients behave abnormally and indulge in unusual sexual practices. Sometimes one person approaches the sex worker and book her but later he would come with four or five persons. They have to put up with all this. (Director of an NGO)

The wider community, health care providers, and the police

The overwhelming majority of the respondents in both categories reported community members as the major source of stigma and discrimination. They feel that they are perceived as immoral or indulging in unnatural behaviour. Men who are engaged in sex work are doubly stigmatized on account of their occupation. Female sex workers reported comparatively more stigma from the women in the community, while *kothis* faced comparatively more stigmatizing behaviour from men in the community. Respondents from both the groups reported that community members assign criminal attributes to them; they are seen as people who will do anything for money, and petty thefts and robbery are frequently attributed to them.

The respondents seek health services from multiple sources. Predominantly respondents in both groups use condom services from the NGOs engaged in HIV prevention work. Some use condoms from government hospitals or ask the client to bring them. Few purchase condoms from shops. General medical services, STI treatment and HIV testing services are used from a mix of public, private and NGO providers. Some seek STI and other treatment from traditional healers and other unqualified practitioners.

Although government hospitals and NGOs are generally more accessible financially, they do not provide adequate services or drugs. Many respondents are therefore forced to make use of private services at a higher cost. Most of the respondents do not reveal their occupation or sexual identity when seeking health care from either government or private hospitals. At times, their identity becomes known, and such respondents report experiences of stigmatizing behaviour and discrimination while seeking medical care. A few respondents also reported discriminatory behaviour from staff of NGOs engaged in HIV prevention work. Men reported that they were degraded and abused, their identity was revealed to others in their community, and they were sometimes denied services and expelled from health care facilities by doctors and hospital staff. Female sex workers reported that they were degraded and criticized, not examined properly, forced to undergo HIV tests, overcharged for services at private hospitals, denied medical services and delivery care, and that their identity was revealed to others in the community.

> *Some of the doctors, when we approach them for treatment, if they know that we are [kothis] they don't touch us and go away from us ordering the [security staff] to send us out.*

> *Without conducting blood test and HIV test doctors do not touch us in hospitals. During delivery time when we want to have hospital delivery, they do not admit us in hospitals for delivery.*

NGO staff and gatekeepers in the sites corroborate such experiences of discrimination. NGO staff reveal that, in some cases, even doctors appointed by NGOs specifically for the purpose of providing treatment to female sex workers and *kothis* discriminate against them.

Significant numbers of respondents from both groups reported discrimination and violence at the hands of the police. Female sex workers reported that they were verbally abused, beaten up, forced to have sex without payment, robbed of their money and other valuables, threatened and harassed by the police. At times, they are arrested and fined when they are caught with a client. Sometimes false cases are foisted on them if the police do not have enough cases registered at the police station. As a female sex worker records:

> *Police people harass us a lot. They beat us very often and keep us in jail... They come to our houses also and without even inquiring they start beating us. They beat me like this many times. Their [officer] had instructed them to beat us whenever they want. It is their wish. They beat and went away.*

Kothis report that the police verbally and physically abuse them, demand bribes and blackmail them with a threat of defaming them in public. Some reported that they were forced to have sex with police personnel. NGO personnel corroborate that abuse and violence of female sex workers and *kothis* by police is widespread:

Police exploit kothis and female sex workers. They use them sexually for themselves and send them to others for personal favours. They take away whatever money female sex workers and kothis are having in the name of bribe for not beating them But, if they find that general population are watching, then they beat them and send them away.

Coping with stigma, discrimination and violence

The majority of the respondents from both groups said that they felt 'sad', 'bad', 'upset' 'scared' or 'ashamed' when faced with stigma and discrimination. Some reported that they felt 'angry', 'depressed or 'helpless'. Some said that they 'felt like dying', a few attempted suicide in an acute reaction to stigma and discrimination, and some said that they felt like giving up sex work.

I feel sad at the discrimination. Sometimes I wonder why I had to do sex work and I feel like dying. (Female sex worker)

When my neighbours spoke ill of me, I felt very bad and consumed pesticide. I had to spend around 10,000 rupees to get treatment and gain consciousness. (Kothi)

Given their reactions to stigma and the fears that dominate their lives, it is apparent that the respondents were under a great deal of stress. They make conscious efforts to reduce and minimize their stress levels. Respondents from both groups reported that they mainly deal with such stress on their own and that they do not receive much support from others. Coping strategies identified by the respondents included: leaving the place when faced with abuse; avoiding perpetrators or situations where there is possibility of getting stigmatized and abused; and not going out alone or going out with peers.

A significant number of the respondents said that they retaliate when faced with stigmatizing behaviour and abuse from the community. This may be through answering them back or abusing the perpetrator. Many try to resist physical abuse from others and fight back. Indulgence in alcohol was a commonly adopted coping mechanism, especially by the female sex workers. Few of the respondents try to cope by sharing their experiences with parents, spouses or partners, friends and peers:

Sometimes when people stigmatize us we will resign everything to God and ignore them thinking that they will only bear the consequences later. Some times I get crazy thoughts. I think that my life has become spoilt and that my children will also be spoilt. I become depressed then and go to movies or consume brandy. (Female sex worker)

The respondents were wary of seeking support from others, fearing further stigmatization and, as such, very few reported having received any active support from others. When they did receive support from others, e.g. peers, gatekeepers, spouses, people in toddy shops, police, neighbours, friends, acquaintances and members of their caste, it consisted of them speaking on behalf of the respondent or coming to their rescue; negotiating, punishing, warning or threatening perpetrators; as well as providing emotional and monetary support.

Some respondents, especially *kothis*, identified themselves with peer groups. Generally *kothi* peer groups are well structured with specific roles for each member. They meet together, attend functions, parties, movies, solicit business and sometimes help each other. Female sex workers have a comparatively lower level involvement in peer groups. Female sex worker peer groups usually consist of a small informal grouping of sex workers working in an area, who get together and talk with each other in the course of work.

Involvement in peer groups may be seen as a coping strategy adopted by the respondents. Respondents, especially *kothis*, expressed a feeling of belonging in peer groups. Many were able to share their grievances with each other and, at times, help each other. Some of them expressed the need for the formation of stronger peer groups for better support. As described above, however, relations between peers are not always easy and, because of lack of trust, these groups can become unstable and disintegrate.

The NGOs working on HIV/AIDS in these sites play an important role in helping respondents cope with stigma. Most of the respondents were willing to disclose their identity to NGO staff and outreach workers. Since the outreach workers were from the key populations themselves, many respondents said that they found such people more accessible. NGO presence has played a significant role in improving awareness regarding STIs and their prevention, and providing access to condom services, STI treatment, HIV testing and, in some cases, general medical treatment. Most of the respondents who were using condoms regularly said that they began regular condom use in the last 6-12 months, which coincides with the time when the NGOs began work.

As a result of the work of the NGOs, many respondents had a high level of expectation from them, especially regarding prevention of abuse and violence experienced by them, provision of alternate employment, and financial and material support. However, most respondents reported that they did not get any such support. Neither did they have much voice or decision making role in the implementation of the programme:

> *The NGO supplies only condoms. They do not provide any help during violence. We can buy condoms outside for one rupee which we can afford. We need help to combat our problems. We can get rid of all these problems if the NGO can provide alternative employment. (Female sex worker)*

Discussion and conclusion

Female sex workers and *kothis* are similar in many ways. Both are powerless, highly marginalized and hidden, while a large section of the male population from the general population accesses them for sexual purposes. Despite the fact that they are accessed by a large number of male clients, our study findings clearly indicate that the experience of stigma is very much part of their lives. Violence and discrimination are all around them, all the time. Whilst there are specific variations in the language and expression of stigma, discrimination and violence, both respondent types appear to suffer equally from their occupation and identity. Both deal with feelings of rejection, degradation, isolation, loss of self-esteem and self-respect, fear and violence. Sex workers and *kothis* are stigmatized because they are poor, low caste, are the locus for enacting gender and masculinity norms, engage in deviant sexual behaviour, and are also seen as transmitters of infections.

Some differences between sex workers and *kothis* that stand out include the fact that sex workers experienced more stigma from their families than did *kothis*, but this could be explained by the fact that more women had told their families about their occupation. Additionally, whilst women had fewer friends but saw them as a source of support in whom they trust and confide, men tended to suffer much stigma from these so-called friends. Similarly, the experience of peer relationships is mixed: on the one hand, they look to their peers for emotional and financial support; at the same time, because of differences in, amongst other things, the kind of sex work in which that are engaged (street or home-based), their looks and their socioeconomic status, jealousies and rivalries, all resulting in mistrust, are widespread.

An issue that has largely remained unaddressed in HIV/AIDS programming relates to the clients of sex workers. Male clients of both female and male sex workers are both the perpetrators of violence, stigma and discrimination and ironically also the potential protectors. HIV prevention programmes in India have systematically targeted sex workers, particularly female sex workers, almost at the exclusion of their clients who constitute an important bridge between sex workers and the general population. Within the categories of men who have sex with men, the majority of the *panthis*, who are exclusively the partners of *kothis*, remain an invisible and hidden group as they are either married or likely to be married in the future. It is this hidden population of male clients who will make a significant difference to prevention and care programmes in the future.

Coping with stigma, discrimination and violence is a complex issue as it often involves individual responses which are frequently associated with individual characteristics, personalities, levels of confidence and self-esteem. A common action thought to assist vulnerable groups to cope with their situation, to build self-confidence and self-esteem as well as trust, is to develop peer support groups and/or collectives. Nevertheless, as has been shown in this study, although they do go some way to providing an answer, because of deep rooted differences, jealousies and rivalries, mistrust often increases and support groups are unsuccessful and disintegrate.

The enabling environment has a clear role to play in assisting members of key populations to cope with stigma, discrimination and violence. The enabling environment in this case ranges from families, to neighbours, peers, police and policy makers. All of these different groups have a specific role at their different levels, and projects need to ensure that either they integrate them into their programmes or they link up with other projects working with one specific group.

As is shown by our study and similar studies elsewhere, stigmatizing attitudes are the reflections of deep rooted and hierarchical social structures. Almost all the female sex worker respondents and most of the male respondents came from a poor socioeconomic background: relatively few were literate, and few reported having had the opportunity to develop any kind of life skills. Although the stigmatizing effects of poverty were reported by both groups of respondents, the burden was seen disproportionately higher in the female sex workers.

Caste related stigma also plays a role in the stigmatization of respondents, especially female sex workers. Stigma and discrimination of lower castes is a condition of life within the Indian cultural milieu and members of lower castes experience a higher level of poverty compared to the upper castes. Women belonging to castes traditionally associated with sex work are further stigmatized.

Within this deep-rooted social structure, the norms of masculinity and gender assist in explaining a large part of the stigma and violence faced by female sex workers and *kothis*. A gender framework and the social construction of masculinity that places men in a more advantageous position than women is at the root of this powerlessness for both the populations. Most female sex workers are pushed into the sex trade by economic deprivation and desertion. This is also true for the majority of *kothis* who belong to a marginalized social and economic class.

The NGOs working with sex workers and *kothis* face the challenge of going beyond HIV/AIDS to work at developing a context specific strategy to organize and empower them. Given the stigmatized and violent context in which these groups exist, condom distribution and STI prevention alone will not be sufficient to bring about changes in the attitudes and behaviours of key stakeholders, including police, clients and sex workers themselves. When sex workers and *kothis* do not wish to reveal their identity, ways must be found to peg the empowerment programme to a larger development programme while, at the same time, ensuring participation of community members, men in general, gatekeepers and police. Where individuals are open about their occupation and identity, they should be brought in as advocates, as peer educators and as advisers.

For *kothis*, the most meaningful sense of empowerment comes from their clients or male partners *(panthis)*. It appears feasible to work with *kothis* and their male partners, whereas for female sex workers the effort has also to focus on developing meaningful collectives. Key in both cases is knowledge and skills to help them deal with day-to-day issues and build a community-based support system.

Programmes that include the wider community are better placed for tackling issues of stigma, discrimination and violence. A focus on the family is also crucial when considering programmatic implications since a supportive and understanding family environment can be seen as a springboard into the community, providing an individual with increased levels of confidence and self-esteem.

stigma, discrimination and violence

References

Ainsworth, M. and M. Over, 'Confronting AIDS: public priorities in a global epidemic'. *A World Bank Policy Research Report*. Washington, DC, Oxford University Press, rev. ed., 1999.

Asthana, Sheena and Robert Oostvogels, 'The social construction of male 'homosexuality' in India: implications for HIV transmission and prevention'. *Social Science and Medicine* vol. 52, no. 5 (2001), p. 707-721.

Bhave, G., C.P. Lindan, E.S. Hudes, S. Desai, U. Wagle, S.P. Tripathi and J.S. Mandel, 'Impact of an intervention on HIV, sexually transmitted diseases, and condom use among sex workers in Bombay, India'. *AIDS* vol. 9, Suppl. 1 (1995), p. S21-30.

Boer, H. and P.A.A. Emons, 'Accurate and inaccurate HIV transmission beliefs, stigmatizing and HIV protection motivation in northern Thailand'. *AIDS Care* vol. 16, no. 2 (2004), p. 167-176.

Brown, L., F. Yokota, Y. Sawadogo and A. Afable, 'Stigma measurement in Africa: a comparative analysis of DHS and BSS Surveys'. 2004. (Forthcoming working paper for MEASURE Evaluation).

Campbell, C. and Z. Mzaidume, 'Grassroots participation, peer education, and HIV Prevention by sex workers in South Africa'. *American Journal of Public Health* vol. 91, no. 12 (2001), p. 1978-1986.

Global HIV Prevention Working Group, 'Access to HIV prevention: closing the gap'. 2003.

Goffman, E., *Stigma: notes on the management of spoiled identity*. New York, NY, Prentice-Hall, 1963.

Herek, G.M. and J.P. Capitanio, 'AIDS stigma and contact with persons with AIDS: effects of direct and vicarious contact'. *Journal of Applied Social Psychology* vol. 27, no. 1 (1997), p. 1-36.

Herek, G., J. Capitanio and K.F. Widaman, 'HIV-related stigma and knowledge in the United States: prevalence and trends, 1991-1999'. *American Journal of Public Health* vol. 92, no. 3 (2002), p. 371-377

Kalichman, S.C. and L. Simbayi, 'Traditional beliefs about the cause of AIDS and AIDS-related stigma in South Africa'. *AIDS Care* vol. 16, no. 5 (2004), p. 572-580.

Khan, Shivananda, 'Masculinities, (homo)sexualities and HIV vulnerability: working with males who have sex with males in India'. London, Naz Foundation International, 2005. <www.nfi.net>

KIT, 'Report of a research workshop on health related stigma and discrimination'. Amsterdam, KIT (Koninklijk Instituut voor de Tropen/Royal Tropical Institute), December 2004.

NACO (National AIDS Control Organization), 'Statewise HIV prevalence (1998-2003)'. New Delhi, NACO, Ministry of Health & Family Welfare, Government of India, 2004.

NACO (National AIDS Control Organization), 'HIV estimates.' New Delhi, NACO, 2003.

Nyblade, L., 'Measuring HIV stigma: existing knowledge, gaps, challenges, and moving Forward'. Soesterberg, Research workshop on health-related stigma and discrimination, 2004.

Ogden, J. and L. Nyblade, 'Common at its core: HIV-related stigma across contexts'. Washington, DC, International Center for Research on Women (ICRW), 2005.

Parker, R. and P. Aggleton, 'HIV and AIDS-related stigma and discrimination: a conceptual framework and implications for action'. *Social Science and Medicine* vol. 57, no. 1 (2003), p. 15-24.

Piot, Peter, 'Panel on exploring the link: HIV/AIDS, stigma, discrimination and racism'. United Nations High Commissioner for Human Rights, 5 September 2001.

Ramasubban, R., 'Patriarchy and the risks of STD and HIV transmission'. In: M. Das Gupta, L. Chen and T. Krishnan, *Women's health in India: risk and vulnerability*. Delhi, Oxford University Press, 1998, p. 212-241.

Rodrigues, J. et al, 'Risk factors for HIV infection in people attending clinics for sexually transmitted diseases in India'. *British Medical Journal* vol. 311, no. 7000 (1995), p. 283-286.

Salunke, S., M. Jagtap, S. Hira, P. Dalal and C. Jagavkar, 'Rapid rise in HIV prevalence among women attending government STD clinic in Mumbai (Bombay), India'. *International Journal of STD & AIDS* vol. 8, no. 4 (1997), p. 280.

Thappa, D.M., S. Singh and A. Singh, 'HIV infection and sexually transmitted diseases in a referral STD centre in south India'. *Sexually Transmitted Infections* vol. 75, no. 3 (1999), p. 191.

UNAIDS, 'Compendium on discrimination, stigmatisation and denial'. Geneva, UNAIDS, 2001.

UNAIDS, 'Epidemiological fact sheet on HIV/AIDS and sexually transmitted diseases'. Geneva, UNAIDS, 2000.

UNAIDS, 'Report on the global AIDS epidemic'. Geneva, UNAIDS, 2004.

UNESCO, 'Towards a handbook for India: a cultural approach to HIV/AIDS prevention and care'. *Studies and Reports, Special Series, no. 5.* Paris, UNESCO, 2001.

USAID, 'Working report measuring HIV stigma: results of a field test in Tanzania'. Washington, DC, USAID, 2005.

Verma, Ravi K. and M. Collumbien, 'Homosexual activity among rural Indian men: implications for HIV prevention'. *AIDS* vol. 18 (2004), p. 1845-1847.

stigma, discrimination and violence

A guide to the bibliography: explanation of the records in the bibliography

The records in the annotated bibliography are listed alphabetically by author, a subject and a geographical index, which give the record number within the bibliography. Each record is complemented by an abstract.

PHOTOCOPYING SERVICES: libraries, organizations as well as individual users from any country in the world may request photocopies of articles and small books (up to 100 pages) included in the bibliography.

Photocopying services for users in developing countries are free-of-charge. Information about charges and library services can be requested at Information and Library Services (ILS).

Please state the KIT Library shelf mark of the book(s), chapter(s) or journal article(s) in your request.

Information and Library Services
KIT (Royal Tropical Institute)
P.O. Box 95001
1090 HA Amsterdam, The Netherlands
Fax: +31 (0)20-6654423
E-mail: library@kit.nl
URL: http://www.kit.nl/ils/

An example of a typical record is shown below:

[1] **004** [2] **Restructuring the health system: experience of advocates for gender equity in Bangladesh**
[3] JAHAN, ROUNAQ. [4] Reproductive Health Matters, (2003)21, p. 183-191, [5] refs [6] ISSN 0968-8080
An analysis of health sector reforms and reform advocates in Bangladesh from 1995-2002 is made. The focus is on the gaps between reform design by advocates and implementation through government- and donor-driven programmes. Advocacy has succeeded in heightening awareness of social and gender inequality and increasing the involvement of women in reform design. However, a government change in 2001 is linked to a weakening of the capacity to implement the reforms, due to a shift in focus and priorities.
Successful continuation of the implementation of reforms is seen to depend on sustained civil society advocacy and alliances with other groups such as the women's movement, in addition to promotion through government channels.
KIT Library shelf mark [7] **D 3099-(2003)21**

1) Record number.

2) Original title.

3) All authors are listed and entered in the Author Index.

4) The reference includes the journal title in full (in italics), the volume number, year of publication (in brackets), issue number, inclusive page numbers as stated in the original document. For monographs, the publisher, place, number of pages and year of publication are given.

5) Summaries, glossaries, indexes, illustrations and literature references are also noted.

6) The bibliographic data conclude with the ISSN or ISBN (if available) of the original document.

7) A unique library code, of the book, chapters or journal articles, available in KIT Library, is given at the end of each record. Please state this shelf mark in your photocopy request. When it concerns an electronic document, the URL is provided, however, photocopies of these documents are also available at KIT Library.

Annotated bibliography

001 Abandoning female genital mutilation/cutting: information from around the world (CD-ROM)
Washington, DC, Population Reference Bureau, 2005
This CD-ROM, in English and in French, is a collection of data and research on female genital mutilation/cutting (FGM/C) from a wide variety of sources. Funded by USAID, this resource is a direct response to the findings of a 2004 survey, undertaken by the Population Reference Bureau with four collaborating partners, in which respondents said that serious information gaps on FGM/C exist. The CD-ROM fills some of these information gaps, particularly where the Internet is an expensive and unreliable method of research, by including material on various approaches used by organizations working toward abandonment of FGM/C, as well as on statistics, training efforts, and policy aspects. This resource is being disseminated to various NGOs and individuals worldwide.
Single copies of the CD-ROM are available free of charge, please contact the Population Reference Bureau at prborders@prb.org

002 Access to quality gender-sensitive health services: women-centred action research
Kuala Lumpur, Asian-Pacific Resource and Research Centre for Women (ARROW), 2003. 147 p.
This publication is the outcome from an action-research project to assess low-income and marginalized women's access to gender-sensitive, quality health services in selected countries. The study aimed to effect changes in the perception of health service providers and in women's knowledge of their rights to quality health services resulting in an improved access and more gender-sensitive provision of health services for women in Asia and Pacific. A participatory methodology and intervention were designed and implemented in cooperation with service providers, women and women's organizations. The main findings are drawn from an analysis of the six case studies of health services conducted in Malaysia, Bangladesh, Philippines, China, Sri Lanka and Pakistan. The book offers insight into experiences of health services and needs as articulated by women themselves and is useful to governments, international institutions and NGOs who are committed to reviewing health programmes for women as recommended by the Fourth World Conference on Women (Beijing).
http://arrow.org.my/images/Women's%20Access%20 Main.pdf (contents)
http://arrow.org.my/images/Women's%20Access%20 Cover%20&%20Table%20of%20Contents.pdf (cover and table of contents) (accessed October 2005)

003 Integration of reproductive health services for men in health and family welfare centers in Bangladesh
AL-SABIR, AHMED; ALAM, MOHAMMED AHSANUL; HOSSAIN, SHARIF MOHAMMED ISMAIL; ROB, UBAIDUR; KHAN, M.E. New York, NY, Population Council, 2004. 38 p.
The Bangladesh national family planning programme introduced in the mid-1970s focused primarily on women. It facilitated women's access to information and medical care, however neglected the medical needs of males. Men tend to visit pharmacies, private practitioners and district hospitals. They seldom take preventive steps and delay seeking help for chronic health problems. A 2-year experimental study at 8 intervention sites and 4 control sites shows that male reproductive health services can easily be integrated within existing family planning and health care delivery systems. Local awareness raising, group discussions and behaviour change communication methods result in increased numbers of male clients seeking help from (usually female-focused) Health and Family Welfare Centres (HFWCs), and also a substantial rise in the number of female clients. Practical training for service providers on male reproductive health problems, reproductive tract infections (RTIs) and sexually transmitted

infections (STIs) is needed to enable the diagnosis and treatment of RTI and STI cases and extra medicines must be supplied. However, the rise in the total number of male and female clients at HFWCs leads to more effective use of resources and a lower cost of treatment per patient.

http://www.popcouncil.org/pdfs/frontiers/FR_Final Reports/Bangladesh_Male%20Involvement.pdf (accessed October 2005)

004 Gender, leprosy and leprosy control: a case study in Plateau State, Nigeria
ALUBO, OGOH. Amsterdam, Royal Tropical Institute (KIT), 2003. 126 p. ISBN 90-6832-718-6
The prevalence of leprosy in Plateau State, Nigeria amounts around 0.61 per 10,000 people, consisting almost equally of men and women. Men tend to suffer more from multibacillary leprosy more than women and have more deformities. Women in the reproductive age group tend to under-report compared to men. Women may be more susceptible to leprosy infection, but have a better immune system. The latter may be temporarily weakened by pregnancy, but it reacts better than with men to BCG immunization. Recognition of early leprosy remains difficult in spite of 40 years of leprosy control. Awareness of and a positive attitude towards biomedical treatment is generally high. Beliefs in supernatural causes of leprosy remain strong, as do misunderstandings concerning its infectiousness, which contribute to stigmatization. Women are more likely to fear domestic stigma, which could lead to divorce and lost access to their children. Men fear community stigma, because of loss of status, respect, income and public rejection as a result of deformities. Case holding in Nigeria is more difficult than case finding, especially relating to men.
KIT Library shelf mark: N 04-288; N 04-300

005 Gender, leprosy and leprosy control: a case study in Rio de Janeiro State, Brazil
ALVEZ MOREIRA, TADIANA M.; VARKEVISSER, CORLIEN M. Amsterdam, Royal Tropical Institute (KIT), 2002. 83 p. ISBN 90-6832-715-1
In Rio de Janeiro State, the male/female ratio among leprosy patients appears to be roughly 1. However, men suffer significantly more from the serious multibacillary form and have more deformities and reactions than women. Growing evidence indicates that hormone levels during women's reproductive years may influence the seriousness and incidence of leprosy. Since 1996, slightly more female than male patients have been registered. This may be linked to the significantly higher level of awareness among women of the increased accessibility of treatment points and of leprosy education campaigns which accompanied the decentralization of services. Socio-cultural factors appear to drive this higher awareness: greater awareness of physical symptoms and worries related to female images of beauty and attractiveness. Women appear to suffer more than men from stigma. Leprosy services are more accessible to women patients through the high level of delivery by female staff (80%), but mis-diagnosis is more likely among women, who experience relatively less easily recognized symptoms. The cure rate is over 80% for both men and women, although women came for treatment less regularly. Stronger counseling and community education is needed to improve case finding and case holding. There are still widely prevalent beliefs that leprosy is incurable and highly infectious.
KIT Library shelf mark: N 03-496; N 03-497

006 Workshop on sexual and bodily rights as human rights in the Middle East and North Africa: summary report
AMADO, LIZ ERCEVIK; ILKKARACAN, PINAR (ed). Istanbul, Women for Women's Human Rights (WWHR) – New Ways), 2004. 21 p.
The workshop was co-organized by Women for Women's Human Rights – New Ways and the Mediterranean Academy of Diplomatic Studies and held at Malta from May 29-June 1, 2003. Sexual and bodily rights should be put on the public agenda in the Middle East and North Africa, in the light of discussions concerning (violations of) human rights, sexuality and gender identity, sexuality and law, and sexuality and sexual health. Biases against work on sexuality declare it either as the promotion of lesbianism or as blasphemy. The issue extends beyond women's sexuality, however, and consideration of male sexuality would be necessary to complete the picture, given that it is linked to constructs of female sexuality. Sexual orientation as a human rights issues has achieved some visibility in the region, and a rising awareness of a need to address homosexuality reveals a significant transformation that is underway. Implementing laws and changing social practices is a major concern. Working with young people is central, and regional and international networking is also essential. Sexuality still remains a taboo in the region and violations of sexual and bodily rights are still prevalent. The issue must be addressed from a holistic perspective, however, since sexuality and

bodily rights are at the core of human rights and must be realized if equality, autonomy and empowerment are to be achieved.
http://iwhc.org/docUploads/Malta%20Summary%20Report.pdf (accessed October 2005)

007 Gender mainstreaming in HIV/AIDS: taking a multisectoral approach
AMARATUNGA, CAROL et al. London, Commonwealth Secretariat, 2002. 164 p. refs. ISBN 0-85092-655-6
The Commonwealth approach to gender mainstreaming is the Gender Management System, a holistic, system-wide approach to bringing a gender perspective to bear in the mainstream of all government policies, plans and programmes. The manual offers a number of case studies from developing and developed countries, which illustrate how programmes that promote HIV prevention by addressing gender and the social and economic factors that increase people's risk of infection are more likely to succeed in changing behaviour. It also contains an extensive list of online resources.
KIT Library shelf mark: N 02-843

008 Annotated bibliography: gender, HIV/AIDS and development
Ottawa, Interagency Coalition on AIDS and Development (ICAD), 2005. 8 p.
One of the most important developments in the global fight against HIV/AIDS is the recognition of the role of gender in fuelling the spread and increasing the burden of the epidemic. This document compiles key online resources that describe the current understanding of, and responses to, the effects of gender on HIV/AIDS at the international level. Resources were selected to provide a balanced approach that addresses both men's and women's concerns, vulnerabilities, challenges, and responses to gender and HIV/AIDS issues. A special focus on gender-based violence is included because of the tremendous impact of sexual violence on risk of HIV infection.
http://icad-cisd.com/pdf/publications/Final_English_AnnoBiblio_GenderHIVAIDS_Dev....pdf (accessed October 2005)

009 Annotated bibliography: selected WHO publications on gender, women and health 1999-2005. Contribution to the 10-Year Review of the Beijing Platform for Action
Geneva, World Health Organization (WHO), 2005. 15 p.
This annotated bibliography provides a selected list of publications produced by the World Health Organization focusing on women and/or gender in the last six years. It also includes a comprehensive list of all publications produced by the Department of Gender, Women and Health. While many more publications specifically related to women and gender have been produced by the organization, (including regional and country-level publications), the aim of this compilation is to reference key global documents. For the sake of brevity, specific references to newsletters, reports of meetings, or country-level analyses have been excluded. Please note that additional information on these and other WHO publications relating to gender, women and health can be found on the official WHO website, www.who.int. This bibliography serves as a follow-up to the 1999 WHO Review of Activities which documented specific programmes, policies and activities undertaken by the organization to implement the Beijing Platform for Action.
http://www.who.int/gender/documents/Annotated%20Bibliography%20green%20A4.pdf (accessed October 2005)

010 Annotated bibliography on gender mainstreaming and analysis resources for health programmers
Washington, DC, Gender and Health Unit, Pan-American Health Organization (PAHO), 2003. 29 p.
This bibliography comprises reports, manuals, guidelines etc. on mainstreaming gender in health projects, programmes and policies. The resources are grouped according to: introductions to gender; gender policies; plans and commitments; gender mainstreaming manuals and guides; gender analysis tools and guides; and gender and specific health topics such as ageing, communicable diseases, reproductive health, and violence and injuries.
http://www.paho.org/English/DPM/GPP/GH/Main streamingBibliography.pdf (accessed October 2005)

011 Re-thinking sexualities in Africa
ARNFRED, SIGNE (ed). *Sexuality, Gender and Society in Africa Research Programme 1.* Uppsala, Nordiska Afrikainstitutet, 2004. 276 p. ISBN 91-7106-513-X
Empirical studies carried out by Europeans and Africans examine the influences of colonialism and Christianity on attitudes to sexuality in African societies, e.g. in Namibia, Senegal and Ghana. Fresh approaches examine the integration of different cultural spaces into changing gender and sexual identities. The cultural meanings of female circumcision, how the relative invisibility of women affects the incidence of HIV/AIDS, and male-female power balances in decision making on childbearing are all considered from a post-colonial point of view. Issues of male and female sexual desire are

analysed in relation to questions of race and politics in South Africa and Mali. Links between female sexuality and social status, and the socioeconomic effects of African women's handling of the culture of silence are studied in the context of feminism and the gender discourse.

KIT Library shelf mark: N 04-279

012 Women of our world 2005
ASHFORD, LORI; CLIFTON, DONNA. Washington, DC, Population Reference Bureau, 2005. 12 p.
Data on demography and reproductive health are presented, broken down by geographic regions and defined according to number of women in total and in different age groups, lifetime births per woman, percentage aged 15-19 giving birth in one year, percentage of married women using contraception, maternal deaths per 100 000, lifetime chance of death from maternal causes, abortion policy per country, percentage of adults aged 15-49 with HIV/AIDS, and percentage of HIV-infected women.

http://www.prb.org/pdf05/WomenOfOurWorld2005.pdf
(accessed October 2005)

013 Female genital mutilation in Upper East region of Ghana: a public health concern
ATINGA, JULIET ALICE. Amsterdam, Royal Tropical Institute (KIT), 2004. 48 p.
Female genital mutilation (FGM) is most prevalent in Ghana in the Upper East Region: about 70% of women aged 15-49 are affected. It is still being practiced, in spite of the increased attention of the international community, health professionals and human rights activists worldwide. The main reasons for its practice relate to social identity, religion, and beliefs concerning hygiene aesthetics, and sexuality. FGM has strong traditional links, and is practiced by members of all religions and levels of education and urbanization. It is essential for community leaders to work with community-based organizations and NGOs if the practice is to be discontinued. There is a need for concerted efforts at national and community levels, and the involvement of men in programmes to eradicate this violent and harmful practice.

KIT Library shelf mark: G 04-111

014 Senegalese grandmothers promote improved maternal and child nutrition practices: the guardians of tradition are not averse to change
AUBEL, JUDI; TOURÉ, IBRAHIMA; DIAGNE, MAMADOU. *Social Science and Medicine* 59(2004)5, p. 945-959, refs. ISSN 0277-9536
In many places, older women play an influential role in domestic maternal and child health. A participatory education project in Senegal encourages grandmothers to promote better nutritional practices surrounding pregnancy and infant feeding. Evaluation data show significant improvements in grandmothers' knowledge of nutritional matters following the intervention. A considerably higher percentage of women of reproductive age (WRA) in villages using the grandmother strategy (91%) report changed behaviour compared to WRA (34%) in villages, which did not engage grandmothers in nutritional education (NE). Participatory communication involves community members, who integrate new, biomedical concepts into traditional approaches using familiar tools such as songs, stories and group discussion. The core of the Senegalese strategy is empowerment, whereby the grandmothers develop their own solutions to problems, based on NE communicated through skilful facilitators. The strategy is thought to bring about longer-lasting changes in behaviour.

KIT Library shelf mark: E 2085-59(2004)5

015 The roles, responsibilities, and realities of married adolescent males and adolescent fathers: a brief literature review
BARKER, GARY; LYRA, JORGE; MEDRADO, BENEDITO. Rio de Janeiro, Instituto Promundo, 2005. 19 p.
Early marriage and fatherhood are relatively uncommon among young men in developing countries, contrary to the situation with young women. Young men are also more likely to continue living with their natal families: 50-80% of men aged 20-24. Nevertheless, the socialization of boys and men and how they treat women is critical to addressing the needs of young married women and adolescent mothers. For this reason, it is important to engage young men in the promotion of better reproductive and sexual health. Some of the issues facing young fathers and married adolescent men include their supposed freedom in choosing partners, sexuality, and reproductive health, the relationship between education, work and family formation, gender-based violence, and HIV/AIDS prevention. Research is lacking on the experiences and roles of adolescent fathers. Recommendations for programmes include the use of role models, training for service providers, workplace-based approaches, involving young fathers and husbands in sexual and reproductive health interventions, training, education and support for young men, and awareness raising for policy makers.

http://www.promundo.org.br/Downloads/PDF/fathers%20&%20married%20adol%20men%205-23-05.pdf
(accessed October 2005)

016 Gender, youth and AIDS
BARROSO, CARMEN. Expert paper prepared for the United Nations Division for the Advancement of Women (DAW) Expert Group meeting 'Achievements, gaps and challenges in linking the implementation of the Beijing Platform for Action and the Millennium Declaration and Millennium Development Goals', Baku, Azerbaijan, 7-10 February 2005. Geneva, United Nations, 11 p.
HIV poses an enormous threat, not only to individual health, but in restricting international development and destabilizing nation-states. The situation has worsened in the last decade. The total number of people living with HIV and AIDS was about 19.5 million in 1995, of which 8 million were women. This rose by the end of 2004 to 40 million people, of whom 20 million are women. The epidemic has a global impact, but reflects regional disparities. Sub-Saharan Africa is the most severely affected. The vulnerability of people in some countries is increased because of factors such as natural disasters, wars, civil conflicts and extreme poverty. According to the U.S. Census Bureau, life expectancies are projected to be 10-14 years lower in Honduras, the Bahamas and Guyana than they would be without AIDS. In spite of advances in treatment and better understanding of the need for a multi-sectoral response, existing measures remain insufficient. Young women are at greatest risk. Rates of HIV infection are more than 3 times higher among women aged 15-24 than among boys of the same age. Gender roles put men at risk also by sanctioning multiple partners and encouraging risk-taking. Interventions must address underlying factors such as low educational levels for women, their relative poverty and limited rights, and vulnerability to violence, because the relationship between HIV prevention and gender equity is reciprocal. The scale-up of prevention and treatment would be cost-effective, since it could reduce costs in later years. Resources should therefore target young people, especially young women.
http://www.un.org/womenwatch/daw/egm/bpfamd2005/experts-papers/EGM-BPFA-MD-MDG-2005-EP.4.pdf (accessed October 2005)

017 Basic indicators for gender equity analysis in health
Washington, DC, Gender, Ethnicity and Health Unit, Pan-American Health Organization (PAHO), 2005. 152 p.
The incorporation of a gender perspective is based on four principles: health, equity, gender, and citizen participation. Gender equity in health is the absence of unfair inequalities, associated with systematic disadvantages for one or other sex. Aside from identity formation, gender is a primary organizing factor of social life. It is central, along with class and race, in the allocation and distribution of resources for health. Detailed indicators for gender equity analysis in health are proposed. Socioeconomic determinants cover demographics, income, education and work, environmental conditions, political and legal dimensions, and health care services financing. Indicators of the state of health cover life expectancy, mortality rates, morbidity, risk behaviours, and sexual and reproductive health. Health care indicators cover access to and use of services, and health care management indicators consider (women's) participation in the labour market, remuneration and the balance of power.
http://www.paho.org/English/AD/GE/basicindicators.pdf (accessed October 2005)

018 Gender and health equity resource guide
BAUME, ELAINE; JUAREZ, MERCEDES; STANDING, HILARY. Brighton, Gender and Health Equity Network, Institute of Development Studies (IDS), 2001. 111 p.
Social inequalities affect who gets ill and what consequences this has in terms of access to and the use of health services. Social policies, therefore, need to respond by incorporating a gender perspective on health issues, as one of the key factors contributing to inequalities in health, education, employment and empowerment. All public health improvements require substantial changes in the wider social context. Equally, all sectors are responsible for the protection and promotion of individuals' health. This resource guide from the Gender and Health Equity Network covers approaches, working methods and practical methodologies, offering a practical map of the information and tools available for incorporation into policies and programmes. Section 1 on institutions mainstreaming gender covers organizational change, donors, agencies, NGOs, national departments and ministries, legal and financial information and sector-wide approaches. Section 2 on implementation covers international gender and health advocacy and health rights. Section 3 provides an overview and examples of tools for gender analysis and incorporation into health care practices. Section 4 reviews resources on the lifespan perspective, and the final section describes issues related to gender and health equity. The objective is to show the relevance of each topic and demonstrate how gender could be achieved, using case studies and examples of good practice

around the world to illustrate the importance of context- and resource-specific strategies.
http://www.ids.ac.uk/ghen/resources/papers/Geneq.pdf (accessed October 2005)

019 Addressing female genital mutilation: challenges and perspectives for health programmes. Part 1: Select approaches
BAUMGARTEN, INGE; KESSLER BODIANG, CLAUDIA. Eschborn, Deutsche Gesellschaft für Technische Zusammenarbeit (GTZ), 2001. 44 p.
The practice of female genital mutilation (FGM), circumcision or genital cutting affects an estimated 130 million girls and women in about 28 countries worldwide. Different approaches to ending the practice are being developed and adapted to suit different contexts. The results of experience with different approaches are summarized for advisers involved in supporting groups working towards abandoning the practice. The approaches have different bases: human rights, legal, health, religion, training of health workers and traditional intermediaries, alternative rituals, behavioural campaigns, social development, and research. Recommendations are presented on the basis of experience with these approaches and the lessons learned. Some successful experiences combine a number of approaches. Possible topics for inclusion in a training curriculum for health workers are listed in Annex 1, as well as two models for the process of individual behaviour change and behaviour adoption in Annex 2. Further elements for the improvement of FGM strategies are offered in a companion publication (Part 2) on GTZ-supported health projects in specific country contexts.
http://www2.gtz.de/dokumente/bib/02-0104.pdf (accessed October 2005)

020 Intergenerational dialogue on gender roles and female genital mutilation in Guinea
BAUMGARTEN, INGE; FINKE, EMANUELA; MANGUET, JEANNE; VON ROENNE, ANNA. *Sexual Health Exchange* 2004, 3/4, p. 17-20. ISSN 1388-3046
An 'intergenerational dialogue' approach to gender, sexual and reproductive health issues including female genital mutilation (FGM) is implemented during a four-day programme of workshops. The workshops initially bring together men and women separately. Local NGO staff members facilitate the process of promoting understanding within groups. The outcomes indicate considerable generational differences, particularly as to pre- and extramarital sexual relationships, HIV/AIDS and condom use, polygamy, the role of fathers, women's marital subjugation, and domestic violence. Dialogue between the sexes reveals an increasing questioning of male behaviour on the part of older women in particular. The programme creates awareness of the need for and benefits of more open communication. A quantitative survey of 40 families of workshop participants and 40 control families in Upper Guinea finds more intergenerational communication among the families of workshop participants. The difficulties encountered relate to cost, because of the length and size of the workshops, and coordination with work or family obligations. Plans for the future include the development of modules to accommodate these conditions. Another key success factor is initial on-the-job training for moderators, because of the importance of their communication skills. Current plans foresee the integration of the intergenerational dialogue method in other sectoral contexts supported by the German Technical Co-operation (GTZ) including health, education and the organizational development of local initiatives.
http://www.kit.nl/ils/exchange_content/assets/images/ Exchange_2004-3-4_English.pdf
KIT Library shelf mark: K 2439-(2004)3/4

021 Beyond the numbers: reviewing maternal deaths and complications to make pregnancy safer
Geneva, World Health Organization (WHO), 2004. 150 p.
Maternal mortality indicators provide an indication of women's status, their access to health care and the adequacy of health care systems, but they are not also easy to ascertain. Additionally, in order to address maternal mortality, countries need information that goes further than merely measuring the extent of the problem. Different approaches include community-based maternal death reviews, facility-based maternal death reviews, confidential enquiries into maternal deaths, surveys of severe morbidity, and clinical audits. Different approaches offer different advantages and disadvantages. There are principles for implementation and key practical issues, which generally apply to these approaches. Sample data collection and analysis forms are provided on a separate CD-ROM as a basis for local adaptation.
http://www.who.int/reproductive-health/publications/ btn/text.pdf (accessed October 2005)

022 The 'so what' report: a look at whether integrating a gender focus into programs makes a difference to outcomes. Interagency Gender Working Group Task Force Report
BOENDER, CAROL; SANTANA, DIANA; SANTILLAN, DIANA; HARDEE, KAREN; GREENE, MARGARET E.; SCHULER, SIDNEY. Washington, DC, Interagency Gender Working Group (IGWG), United States Agency for International Development (USAID), 2004. 86 p. Although women's empowerment seems obviously linked to health and population outcomes, evidence of the links would strengthen the argument for the integration of a gender perspective in health programmes. Nearly 400 interventions have therefore been assessed by the IGWG Task Force to establish their effect. Twenty-five of them are highlighted as examples of programmes that integrate gender. The programmes examined address four reproductive health issues: maternal morbidity and mortality, unintended pregnancy, STIs/HIV, and quality of care. Many interventions have documented effects in more than one of these areas. Interventions are divided into three types: those that exploit gender inequalities, that accommodate gender differences, or that transform gender norms to promote equity. Some innovative programmes accommodate gender differences to achieve short-term results, while seeking to transform gender norms in the long-term. Among the interventions promoting gender equity, more showed results in STI/HIV prevention than in other health areas.
http://www.prb.org/pdf04/TheSoWhatReport.pdf (accessed October 2005)

023 Improving the health sector response to gender based violence: a resource manual for health care professionals in developing countries
BOTT, SARAH; GUEDES, ALESSANDRA; CLARAMUNT, MARIA CECILIA; GUEZMES, ANA. International Planned Parenthood Federation/Western Hemisphere Region (IPPF/WHR), 2004. 229 p.
Based on the experiences of an IPPF/WHR regional initiative to integrate services for victims of gender-based violence into reproductive health programmes, this manual provides tools and guidelines for programme managers working in developing countries. Topics include: planning a programme, implementing routine screenings, providing specialized and emergency services, building reference networks, and legal advocacy. Also included are practical tools to determine provider attitudes to gender-based violence, establish support groups, establish legal definitions and responsibilities, and monitor the quality of care. The manual is also available on CD-ROM.
http://www.ippfwhr.org/publications/download/mono graphs/GBV_Manual_E.pdf (accessed October 2005)

024 Gender, leprosy and leprosy control: a case study in the Far West and Eastern development regions, Nepal
BURATHOKI, KAMALA; et al. Amsterdam, Royal Tropical Institute (KIT), 2004. 120 p. ISBN 90-6832-716-X
The prevalence of leprosy in Nepal is the fifth highest in the world (3.4 per 10,000 of the population), although it has decreased considerably since 1994. More men than women report for treatment, although the ratios are also decreasing over time. Irrespectively of the male/female ratio, significantly more men than women in Eastern Nepal suffer from multibacillary (MB) leprosy and from the deformities associated with MB. There was no significant gender difference in the incidence of MB in the Far West. An important factor contributing to this difference is the delay in reporting for treatment, which was around 10 years for men and 12 for women in the Far West, seven to eight years higher than in other districts. Social and service factors are seen as being responsible for the gender difference, namely lack of education and more traditional beliefs concerning the causes of leprosy, as well as less mobility, decision making power and access to money. Women over 45 tend to be illiterate and more traditionally oriented, thus less likely to believe in medical treatment and the possibility of cure. Fear of stigma results in secrecy. Improved accessibility following decentralization in 1999 has benefited women, but services need more trained female health workers, especially in remote areas, to overcome privacy issues.
KIT Library shelf mark: N 04-1781; N 04-1792

025 Bureau for Global Health strategy for female genital cutting (FGC) (FY 2004-FY 2006)
Washington, DC, Bureau for Global Health, United States Agency for International Development (USAID), 2004. 29 p.
The Bureau for Global Health of the United States Agency for International Development (USAID/GH) is committed to abandonment of the practice of female genital cutting (FGC). A 3-year strategy (2004-2006) aims to achieve the intermediate results of an improved enabling environment and improved quality and effectiveness of community-based FGC abandonment activities. USAID/GH abandonment

activities are locally driven and culturally appropriate, with maximum community-level participation. The focus is on gender and social equity, including women's empowerment and the involvement of men in the process of change. Coordination between donors and governments is sought, as well as efforts to integrate best practices with other initiatives. Key themes are the standardization of training and other materials, expansion and institutionalization at country level, development of successful models in focus countries, research, and the monitoring and evaluation of activities. The strengthening of existing linkages at service delivery, country, agency coordination and USAID unit levels support implementation. Estimated funding for the strategy totals US$5,730,000 over the 3-year period. Funding each year builds on existing programmes, and new initiatives focus on the high priority countries Egypt, Ethiopia, Eritrea, Mali, Guinea, Senegal, Djibouti and Sudan. They are selected according to prevalence, health consequences, donor and local government support, and mission involvement.

http://www.dec.org/pdf_docs/PDACD588.pdf (accessed October 2005)

026 A handbook for advocacy in the African human rights system: advancing reproductive and sexual health
CARBERT, ANNE; STANCHIERI, JULIE; COOK, REBECCA J. Nairobi, Ipas African Regional Office/Ipas Kenya, 2002
The African Charter on Human and Peoples' Rights also relates to reproductive and sexual health rights. Its function and purpose is explained in a manual describing the context of reproductive and sexual health in Africa. The manual includes basic texts such as the African Charter and its draft protocols, regional declarations relating to women's rights, selected African Commission resolutions and national and Commission case law relevant to reproductive and sexual health rights, and international human rights documents relevant to the interpretation of the African Charter rights.

http://www.ipas.org/publications/en/african_advocacy_handbook/handbook_advocacy_african_ch1-6.pdf (chapter 1-6, 78 p.) (accessed October 2005)
http://www.ipas.org/publications/en/african_advocacy_handbook/handbook_advocacy_african_ch7.pdf (chapter 7, 48 p.) (accessed October 2005)
http://www.ipas.org/publications/en/african_advocacy_handbook/handbook_advocacy_african_ch8-10.pdf (chapter 8-10, 58 p.) (accessed October 2005)
http://www.ipas.org/publications/en/african_advocacy_handbook/handbook_advocacy_african_resources.pdf (resources, 22 p.) (accessed October 2005)

027 A manual for integrating gender into reproductive health and HIV programs: from commitment to action
CARO, DEBORAH; SCHUELLER, JANE; RAMSEY, MARYCE; VOET, WENDY. Washington, DC, Interagency Gender Working Group (IGWG), United States Agency for International Development (USAID) Bureau for Global Health, 2003. 71 p.
This reference manual is a companion to the Guide for incorporating gender considerations in USAID's family planning and reproductive health request for proposals and request for applications. It can be used at any stage of a programme from design to implementation and evaluation. Providing information on how to integrate gender concerns into programmes, it enables the development of more effective programmes that meet the needs of participants. Implementers of reproductive health-HIV/AIDS programmes can improve the quality of services and make programmes sustainable. The intention is to better inform and empower clients, improve couple communications, improve utilization of services, create synergies across sectors and broaden the impact of development programmes. By integrating gender concerns, specific outcomes can also be achieved such as improved contraceptive prevalence, reduced HIV transmission, reduced fertility, less violence against women and decreased maternal mortality. The manual can be adapted to suit users' specific priorities, scope and resources. A step-by-step approach with case studies allows programme managers to incorporate individual or multiple elements, and illustrates different ways in which the elements can be incorporated in their programmes.

http://www.prb.org/pdf/ManualIntegrGendr.pdf (accessed October 2005)

028 An assessment of the alternative rites approach for encouraging abandonment of female genital mutilation in Kenya
CHEGE, JANE NJERI; ASKEW, IAN; LIKU, JENNIFER. New York, NY, Population Council, 2001. 56 p.
An alternative rite (AR) of passage programme has been implemented in five districts in Kenya since 1996, in an effort to eradicate the practice of female genital mutilation (FGM). Girls who adopt the AR receive preliminary family life education, which affects their awareness and knowledge of reproductive health. It also generates more positive gender attitudes and higher levels of awareness that FGM contravenes human rights. However, it also appears to generate less positive attitudes towards family

gender and health: policy and practice

planning among unmarried partners and adolescents, including condom use. The process of behavioural change has been influenced by sensitization activities by the Maendeleo Ya Wanawake Organization (MYWO), with technical assistance from the Program for Appropriate Technology in Health (PATH), preceding and accompanying the AR. Other influences have also been observed, specifically that of certain churches and individuals who believe that FGM should be discontinued. The contribution of an AR towards discontinuing the practice depends on the socio-cultural context. Successful implementation of the AR approach in other contexts requires understanding of the cultural role of public ceremonies, in particular, and assessment as to the best format for a ritual that would support those who decide to abandon FGM.
http://www.popcouncil.org/pdfs/frontiers/FR_Final Reports/Kenya_FGC.pdf (accessed October 2005)

029 Closing the gap on sexual and reproductive health and rights in the enlarged European Union
Warsaw, Federation for Women and Family Planning, Secretariat ASTRA Network, 2004. 15 p.
Significant differences continue to grow between east and west within Europe in terms of sexual and reproductive health and rights (SRHR). Growing conservative and religious influences limit sex education and access to contraceptives. In some countries, abortion is used as the only available means of fertility control. In practice, legal abortion services are not accessible, resulting in illegal and unsafe abortions. Additionally, the incidence of STIs including HIV/AIDS has increased considerably in some Central and Eastern European countries. The EU has recognized the need for an effective approach to SRHR to reduce inequalities between new and old EU member states. Recommendations include the development of explicit multi-sectoral approaches, ensuring access to affordable SRHR services and modern family planning methods and extending the existing EU gender equality policies and programmes to SRHR.
http://www.astra.org.pl/eu_report_gap.htm (accessed October 2005)

030 Health, rights and realities: an analysis of the ReproSalud Project in Peru
COE, ANNA-BRITT. Takoma Park, MD, Center for Health and Gender Equity (CHANGE), 2001. 44 p. refs
The ReproSalud project focuses on training community-based organizations (CBOs) and individual women to advocate for health service improvements. It encourages women to confront

barriers against decision making and action for reproductive health. The strategies used by ReproSalud differ from conventional programmes in that it works to create greater equity, increase women's decision making and economic power, and increase the capacity among CBOs to promote effective changes in the health care system to meet women's needs, and ensure accountability of government health programmes. There are signs that the project is making significant advances, although it has encountered constraints. There is a lack of political commitment, and disagreement within many institutions as to the effectiveness of different programmes. Greater capacity and knowledge about reproductive health and rights is needed among administrators and service providers. The project provides lessons for the international community, although it cannot be expected to provide the sole solution for improved reproductive health.
KIT Library shelf mark: Br N 01-1856

031 Reproductive health and human rights: integrating medicine, ethics, and law
COOK, REBECCA J.; DICKENS, BERNARD M.; FATHALLA, MAHMOUD F. Oxford, Clarendon, 2003. 554 p. ISBN 0-19-924133-3
Part 1 one sets out the elements of the medical health care system, and the ethical, legal and human rights dimensions of reproductive and sexual health. It goes on to analyse 15 representative case studies drawn from different regions of the world and experiences that women frequently face. The medical background and the ethical, legal and human rights aspects of each case are examined, charting options for response at the levels of clinical care and health system development. In part 2 ways are suggested to address the social factors that create disadvantage and distress. The final part contains data and sources, including tables on national data on fertility rates, contraceptive use, maternal health status and services, and HIV/AIDS prevalence, as well as on estimated prevalence on of female genital mutilation, and data on abortion mortality and complications.
KIT Library shelf mark: N 04-259

032 Advancing safe motherhood through human rights
COOK, REBECCA J.; DICKENS, BERNARD M. Geneva, World Health Organization (WHO), 2001. 176 p.
Governments are obliged under law to implement human rights in compliance with international treaties. Several human rights established in national laws can be applied to further safe

motherhood, even if they do not specifically focus on maternal health. A large majority of the deaths and complications relating to pregnancy and childbirth occur in developing countries; many of them could be prevented by cost-effective health interventions. Different categories of rights could be applied to relieve the causes of maternal mortality and morbidity. Strategies for the application of human rights are proposed to ensure free choice of maternity and provision of health services and the conditions necessary for safe motherhood. The strategies range from education and training to the negotiation of improved services, and procedures to enforce accountability for safe motherhood.
http://www.who.int/reproductive-health/publications/ RHR_01_5_advancing_safe_motherhood/advancing_safe _motherhood_through_human_rights.pdf (accessed October 2005)

033 Realizing rights: transforming approaches to sexual and reproductive well-being
CORNWALL, ANDREA; WELBOURN, ALICE (eds). London, Zed, 2003. 322 p. refs. ISBN 1-85649-969-3
Innovative programmes in Nigeria, Gambia, South Africa and Brazil have helped to create public awareness of sexual and reproductive health (SRH) issues, especially those affecting women living with HIV and AIDS. Realizing rights calls for strategies that empower people, and also engage with those who put obstacles in the way of change. The case studies therefore focus on key areas that are common to many programmes: identifying and voicing silenced concerns; challenging restrictive norms and values; empowering people and encouraging them to take responsibility for their own SRH; and improving the skills, accountability and responsiveness of service providers and project workers. Participation in these approaches has helped to improve the quality of information and make interventions more appropriate to real situations. It has also helped to bridge the gap between service providers and users.
KIT Library shelf mark: P 03-104

034 Transforming health systems: gender and rights in reproductive health. A training curriculum for health programme managers
COTTINGHAM, JANE; RAVINDRAN, T.K. SUNDARI (ed.). Geneva, Family and Community Health, Department of Reproductive Health and Research, World Health Organization (WHO), 2001. refs. 492 p.
This comprehensive training manual for use with health managers, planners, policy makers and others with responsibilities in reproductive

health includes six modules with case studies and exercises, containing integrated gender and rights articles and covering wide-ranging aspects of reproductive health from maternal mortality to dealing with HIV/AIDS and sexual violence. A gender module introduces the concept of gender as a social construct. It clarifies the differences between gender and sex and discusses the implications of a gender-based division of labour. Implementation of gender mainstreaming and clarification of the links between gender and health conclude the model. The second module introduces social determinants. It discusses how inequities in health result from unequal access to power and resources, and discusses the links between gender and other determinants. The Rights module provides the knowledge needed to apply a human rights framework to the analysis and implementation of reproductive and sexual health policies and programmes. The Evidence module provides training on health research from statistics to measurement and evaluation tools. In the Policy module, the emphasis is on building confidence and the ability to make change happen. The Health systems module discusses the why and how of health reforms and their implications for equity and gender equality. A closing module includes a consolidation exercise and formal closure.
KIT Library shelf mark: U 02-60

035 Abandoning female genital cutting: prevalence, attitudes, and efforts to end the practice
CREEL, LIZ. Washington, DC, Population Reference Bureau, 2001. 37 p.
Female genital cutting (FGC) is a cultural, rather than religious or ethnic practice. National prevalence ranges from 18% in one country to 90% or more in others. It is in decline among younger women in some countries, while in others there has been almost no change over time. FGC abandonment approaches require strong institutions to implement programmes at national, regional and local levels, as well as committed governmental support, inclusion of FGC issues in national health and development programmes, trained health providers, coordination with NGOs and advocacy for programme support and public education. The most successful programmes have been community-based projects for behaviour change using one or more of five approaches. These include integration into initiatives focusing on women's empowerment and collective participation in decision making, development alternative rituals, social marketing to involve community power-holders, and establishing role

models. The Tostan experience in Senegal, for example, shows that collective agreement prevents social stigmatism that might result in girls becoming unmarriageable as a result of stopping FGC. Recommendations are offered for policy makers and programme managers to help create a supportive environment for community-based programmes.
http://www.measurecommunication.org/pdf/Abandoning FGC_Eng.pdf (accessed October 2005)

036 Critical areas, issues and topics in sexual and reproductive health indicator development: an annotated bibliography

New York, NY, International Planned Parenthood Federation/Western Hemisphere Region (IPPF/WHR), and Ford Foundation, 2002. 64 p.
The Reproductive Health Affinity Group, a learning network, established (among other task forces) a Committee on Reproductive Health Indicators. Indicators are needed to measure progress on sexual and reproductive health and rights, and have been developed by major international and local, governmental and non-governmental organizations. Indicators on sexual and reproductive health cover family planning, safe motherhood, abortion, reproductive tract infections/sexually transmitted infections, HIV/AIDS, youth, male involvement and sexuality. Indicators for women's empowerment cover gender equity, rights, education, and violence against women. Indicators for related socioeconomic development areas cover the social context/culture, health sector reform, and migration. Guidelines on indicator development and the importance of both quantitative and qualitative methods are discussed.
http://www.ippfwhr.org/publications/download/mono graphs/srh_indicators_eng.pdf (accessed October 2005)

036a Issue paper on gender and health

DASGUPTA, JASHODHARA; APPEL, MARGUERITE; MUKHOPADHYAY, MAITRAYEE. KIT Development Policy and Practice, March 2004, 48 p.
This paper has been prepared to provide insights into the current state of the debate around gender and health and how the neglect of social inequalities in health and gender power relations can greatly increase vulnerability to ill health and HIV/AIDS. It examines how differences in health status for men and women are not merely biological but fundamentally affected by the social, political and economic forces that shape their lives, in particular the unequal gender power relations. It reveals growing evidence that the range of inequalities, disempowerment and lack of entitlements to decision making power

have contributed significantly to the rampant spread of HIV/AIDS amongst populations who are socially and economically marginalized. It is concluded that since inequalities of power and the lack of rights fundamentally affect equitable health outcomes and are driving the HIV/AIDS pandemic, the promotion and protection of rights should constitute a central part of the response to reduce vulnerability. Emphasized is the critical role active social society constituencies can play in exercising political pressure around the issue of gender equitable approached in public policy.
For a digital copy of this publication, please send an e-mail to: m.valk@kit.nl

037 HIV/AIDS and reproductive health: sensitive and neglected issues. A review of the literature: recommendations for action

DE BRUYN, MARIA. Chapel Hill, NC, Ipas, 2005. 95 p.
Some issues relating to the reproductive health of women living with HIV/AIDS have not yet been given sufficient attention. The main focus of research and programmes in the 1990s was on the prevention of perinatal transmission of HIV, while issues relating to hormonal contraceptive use and abortion have been neglected. This updated literature review addresses provision of contraceptive information for HIV-positive people, HIV counselling and testing during antenatal care and labour before childbirth, options for parenting, and abortion-related care.
http://www.ipas.org/publications/en/HIVLITREV_E05_ en.pdf (accessed October 2005)

038 Reproductive rights for women affected by HIV/AIDS? A project to monitor Millennium Development Goals 5 and 6

DE BRUYN, MARIA. Chapel Hill, NC, Ipas, 2005. 100 p.
To make MDGs 5 and 6 more relevant to the daily work of organizations working for the benefit of women affected by HIV/AIDS, Ipas took the lead in a partnership that developed a resource called: Fulfilling reproductive rights for women affected by HIV: a tool for monitoring achievement of Millennium Development Goals. The monitoring tool suggests benchmarks that can be used to assess steps towards achieving MDGs 5 and 6. In 2005, six organizations partnered with Ipas in trying out the monitoring tool as a data-collection method: Fundación de Estudio e Investigación de la Mujer (FEIM) did so in Argentina, the Gender AIDS Forum in South Africa, the International Community of Women Living with HIV/AIDS in Lesotho and Swaziland, de Encuentro de la Comunidad, A.C. in Mexico, and Women Fighting AIDS in Kenya. Each

partner prepared its own project report and disseminated their findings independently. Ipas prepared this report, which summarizes the overall project, describes how the monitoring tool was used and outlines the main findings presented by the individual organizations. It also includes recommendations regarding use of the monitoring tool and the particular needs that must be addressed in fulfilling the reproductive rights of women affected by HIV/AIDS.

http://www.ipas.org/publications/en/MDGRR_E05_en.pdf (accessed October 2005)

039 Violence, pregnancy and abortion: issues of women's rights and public health. A review of worldwide data and recommendations for action
DE BRUYN, MARIA. Chapel Hill, NC, Ipas, 2003. 82 p.
Surveys indicate that 12-25% of women suffer an attempted or completed rape on at least one occasion. Homeless women and those living with civil unrest, conflict and war are at greatest risk. Women of reproductive age face the most consequences because of the possibility of fatal and non-fatal outcomes: murder and suicide, AIDS and maternal mortality; unwanted pregnancy, miscarriage and stillbirth, unsafe abortion, and long-term consequences for mental and physical health. The links between violence, pregnancy and abortion as yet receive insufficient attention. Following an overview of the context and manifestations of the problem, the review assesses what can and needs to be done, with suggestions for action and appendices including human rights instrument citations, questions to guide health workers, and resources available via the Internet.

http://www.ipas.org/publications/en/violence_against_women/violence_womens_rights_en.pdf (accessed October 2005)

040 Gender or sex: who cares? Skills-building resource pack on gender and reproductive health for adolescents and youth workers, with a special emphasis on violence, HIV/STIs, unwanted pregnancy and unsafe abortion
DE BRUYN, MARIA; FRANCE, NADINE. Chapel Hill, NC, Ipas, 2001. 96 p. ISBN 1-882220-26-9
This resource pack provides complementary sexual and reproductive health (SRH) training materials for adolescents and youth workers. It offers a participatory tool for workshops on how to differentiate gender from sex and show how gender affects SRH. Homework assignments, background materials and additional exercises are included. The content is based on the assumption that adolescents need to be equipped to challenge gendered norms and stereotypes,

which can increase SRH risks. It addresses the interaction of gender with economics, age, power and culture on an individual level.

http://www.ipas.org/publications/en/GENDERSEX_E01_en.pdf (accessed October 2005)

041 Transforming health systems to strengthen implementation of the Beijing Platform for Action and the Millennium Development Goals
DE PINHO, HELEN. Expert paper prepared for the United Nations Division for the Advancement of Women (DAW) Expert Group meeting 'Achievements, gaps and challenges in linking the implementation of the Beijing Platform for Action and the Millennium Declaration and Millennium Development Goals', Baku, Azerbaijan, 7-10 February 2005. 15 p.
The Millennium Development Goals provide an opportunity to review understanding of health systems and their role in contributing to achievement of health goals. Health systems play an important role in the experience of poverty, with the potential as a core social institution that shapes society to redefine this experience. Obligations and commitments to improve women's health have been defined in CEDAW and the Beijing Platform for Action, yet improvement is slow, even regressive in places. Of the approx. 530,000 maternal deaths that occur each year, for example, a disproportionate number occur among the poor. Differences between low-income countries indicate that political commitment is necessary to ensure the successful implementation of programmes for the improvement of maternal health. Sexual and reproductive health information and services must be universally accessible if maternal deaths are to be reduced, and sexual and reproductive health improved. In many cases, broader social factors that must be addressed by other sectors are also influenced by (and influence) health issues, since women's empowerment and increased financial stability would support decision making and access to health care. A shift in the approach to health systems would establish health care as a human right, accessible to all, making delivery a duty of the state. At every level of strategies to improve child, maternal and reproductive health, the balance of power must be challenged and balanced in order to transform health systems.

http://www.un.org/womenwatch/daw/egm/bpfamd2005/experts-papers/EGM-BPFA-MD-MDG-2005-EP.10.pdf (accessed October 2005)

042 Report of experts consultative meetings, Cape Town, South Africa, 21-25 April, 2003: Initiative for Sexual and Reproductive Rights in Health Reforms
DE PINHO, HELEN. Johannesburg, Women's Health Project, University of Witwatersrand, 2003. 45 p.
The goal of the initiative is to improve sexual and reproductive rights and health by increasing knowledge of the role of health sector reform. The aims of the expert consultations were to identify gaps in current understanding and to identify useful lessons that could contribute to advocacy and NGO capacity building. Feedback and insights are provided on health financing, the public/private mix, methodologies for priority-setting, health service decentralization, the integration of services and health service accountability.
http://www.wits.ac.za/whp/rightsandreforms/docs/ExpertConsultationMeetingR.pdf (accessed October 2005)

043 Gender, health and globalization: a critical social movement perspective
DESAI, MANISHA. *Development* 47(2004)2, p. 36-42, refs. ISSN 1011-6370
Focusing on the international women's health movement, it is argued that changing gender relations have engendered the discourse of global health and raised the particular concern of women's health to the forefront of discussions about health. At the same time, the globalization of health and disease has also changed gender relations that have led to community level changes in norms and practices that reproduce gender inequalities.
KIT Library shelf mark: H 1000-47(2004)2

044 The TOSTAN Program: evaluation of a community based education program in Senegal
DIOP, NAFISSATOU J.; FAYE, MODOU MBACKE; MOREAU, AMADOU; CABRAL, JACQUELINE; BENGA, HELENE; CISSE, FATOU; MANE, BABACAR; BAUMGARTEN, INGE; MELCHING, MOLLY. New York, NY, Population Council, 2004. 51 p.
This report evaluates results of a survey of villages in the Kolda region of Senegal, where the NGO TOSTAN ran basic education programmes. Modules cover hygiene, problem-solving, women's health and human rights, and the emphasis is on enabling participants to find their own solutions through more effective analysis of their situation. The programme is part of a movement to discourage female genital cutting (FGC). The targeted participants were mostly women. Testing of the impact of the programme on behaviour with regard to FGC was assessed primarily by the proportion of respondents' daughters aged 0-10 whose parents reported they had undergone FGC. The evaluation indicates a greater increase of awareness of human rights, gender-based violence and FGC among participants in the villages where intervention occurred, compared to a comparison group of similar villages. Women's knowledge increased more than men's, except regarding sexually transmitted infection/HIV. Diffusion of information works well, with knowledge increasing on most indicators among other men and women within the villages besides those who participated in the programme. There is a dramatic decrease in approval of FGC and fewer women want their daughters to undergo FGC in the future. The report documents a substantial impact on women's and men's well being, and sees an extension of the programme as potentially beneficial.
http://www.popcouncil.org/pdfs/frontiers/FR_Final Reports/Senegal_Tostan%20FGC.pdf (accessed October 2005)

045 Health and the Millennium Development Goals
DODD, REBECCA. Geneva, World Health Organization (WHO), 2005. 84 p.
The report presents data on progress on the health goals and targets and looks beyond the numbers to analyse why improvements in health have been slow and to suggest what must be done to change this. It points to weak and inequitable health systems as a key obstacle, including particularly a crisis in health personnel and the urgent need for sustainable health financing. Building up and strengthening health systems is vital if more progress is to be made towards the Millennium Development Goals (MDGs). Unless urgent investments are made in health systems, current rates of progress will not be sufficient to meet most of the MDGs. Key recommendations include to strengthen health systems and ensure they are equitable; to ensure that health is prioritized within overall development and economic policies; and to develop health strategies that respond to the diverse and evolving needs of countries.
http://www.who.int/mdg/publications/mdg_report/en/index.html (accessed October 2005)

046 Including gender in health planning: a guide for regional health authorities
DONNER, LISA. Winnipeg, Prairie Women's Health Centre of Excellence, 2003. 25 p.
Case studies carried out in Manitoba, Canada on mental health and diabetes provide insight into

the practical application of gender-based analysis. When considered from a gendered perspective, for example, women are apparently at greater risk for depression than men, while more men in Manitoba are likely to commit suicide than women. However, factors other than gender alone are necessary to obtain useful information. When gender, age and aboriginal ancestry are taken into account, it can be seen than aboriginal men and women bear a greater burden of illness than other Canadians. They are more like to suffer from chronic diseases, and are for instance at much greater risk of developing diabetes than other Manitobans. The conclusion drawn from these studies is that gender-based analysis aids the health planning process by providing Regional Health Authorities with information that allows priority to be given to areas when gender-sensitive interventions will make a difference.
http://www.pwhce.ca/pdf/gba.pdf (accessed October 2005)

047 **Women and primary health care reform: a discussion paper**
DONNER, LISA; PEDERSON, ANN. Paper prepared for the National workshop on women and primary health care, February 5-7, 2004, Winnipeg, Manitoba
The 1978 WHO Alma Ata Declaration defines primary health care as an essential part of a country's health system, which should be universally accessible and affordable. It is stated to constitute the first element of a continuing health care process, and to include prevention, health promotion, and curative and rehabilitation services. The women's health movement greatly contributed in setting this direction in policy, taking health care approaches into the political domain through an understanding of the need for social and economic changes to bring about gender equity. Primary health care reform initiatives in Canada have been underway for decades, and reflect larger trends towards the commodification of health and health services. None of the reform initiatives dating from the 1960s and 70s have led to major changes, which is still predominantly delivered by doctors on a fee-for-service basis. Health care reform initiatives in Canada do not recognize the importance of gender in primary health care, not the contribution of the women's health movement to its reform.
http://www.cewh-cesf.ca/PDF/health_reform/primary_reform.pdf

048 **Increasing contraceptive use in rural Pakistan: an evaluation of the Lady Health Worker Programme**
DOUTHWAITE, MEGAN; WARD, PATRICK. *Health Policy and Planning* 20(2005)2, p. 117-123 ISSN 0268-1080
Contraceptive use in Pakistan has more than doubled since 1990. The change is attributed to the introduction of the Lady Health Worker (LHW) programme, which provides doorstep primary health care through community-based workers. The programme is part of a Five-Year Plan aimed at increasing access to basic family planning and primary health care, particularly in rural areas. LHWs deliver services related to maternal and child health and treat minor ailments and injuries. They are trained to identify more serious cases and refer them to health professionals. Observers suggest that the LHW programme may help to maintain social barriers that restrict women's mobility. However, they provide women with a choice, and help to achieve family planning goals. LHWs are a cost-effective method of ensuring a sustainable mix of reproductive health services.
KIT Library shelf mark: E 2772-20(2005)2

049 **Gender and health sector reform: a literature review and report from a workshop at Forum 7**
DOYAL, LESLEY. Geneva, Global Forum for Health Research, 2004. 30 p. ISBN 2-940286-28-0
This resource briefing offers an overview of the existing evidence base relating to gender and health sector reform. It begins by examining the different components of these reform processes and why they might have different implications for women and for men. This will reflect both the different biological needs of the two sexes and also the influence of social or gender differences between women and men on health care needs and on access to services and their quality. While available evidence on different aspects of health care will be mentioned, the review will pay particular attention to sexual and reproductive services.
http://www.globalforumhealth.org/filesupld/Gender%20and%20Health%20Sector%20Reform.pdf (accessed October 2005)

050 **Gender equity and public health in Europe: a discussion document**
DOYAL, LESLEY. Paper prepared for the Gender Equity Conference, Dublin, September 2000
In spite of the increasing debate on the links between gender and health, little attention has been given to the development of public health policies in the European Union. There is potential for greater integration of gender equity and

public health policies in Europe with the launch of a new Public Health Programme. Strategy development needs to be based on understanding of the impact of sex and gender on health patterns in the member states. Gender equity in health matters cannot be focused on equalizing longevity or health outcomes because of genetic and biological differences. However, many health problems are not related to specific biological characteristics. Gender inequalities often prevent women from realizing their potential for health. Realistic strategies should therefore ensure that men and women have equal access to health resources. Gender sensitive methods of data collection need to be addressed as well as a gender bias in health research.

http://www.eurohealth.ie/gender/section3.htm (accessed October 2005)

051 Gender equity in health: debates and dilemmas
DOYAL, LESLEY. *Social, Science and Medicine* 51(2000)6, p. 931-939 ISSN 0277-9536
Debates in the late 90s (UN Conferences in Cairo and Beijing) revealed different perceptions of gender equity on the part of traditionalists, feminist radicals and gender radicals. The definition of what is meant by gender equality therefore requires clarification if it is to lead to an equitable distribution of health services. This in turn necessitates identification of the similarities and differences of men and women's health needs, and analysis of the gendered obstacles encountered in accessing resources. The article explores both the biological (sex) and social (gender) aspects of differences. Sex differences are examined in reproductive health care, longevity issues, HIV/AIDS and a number of other health problems. Gender aspects are considered in the context of household and domestic labour responsibilities, breadwinning labour and civil duties; differences in the value and reward assigned to things defined as 'male' or 'female' and the impact this has on the health of men and women. The article proposes an agenda for change that includes policies to ensure equal access to appropriate health care, the reduction of gender inequalities and a loosening of gender role definitions. In conclusion, the paper looks at the potential dilemmas to be confronted in the process of implementation of policies towards achieving gender equity.

KIT Library shelf mark: E 2085-51(2000)6

052 Gender, health and the Millennium Development Goals: a briefing document and resource guide
DOYAL, LESLEY. Geneva, Global Forum for Health Research, 2005. 32 p. ISBN 2-940286-33-7
The document begins with a brief account of the emergence of the Millennium Development Goals (MDGs) and their links to wider health and gender issues. This is followed by a review of some of the major criticisms of the goals from an equity perspective. Section 2 explores the links between gender and the health-related MDGs and the implications of these for research priorities. Section 3 outlines some of the gender issues related to the 'MDG-plus' approach adopted at Forum 8. The document will draw throughout on presentations from Forum 8 and from Forums 6 and 7 where many of these questions were also debated.

http://www.globalforumhealth.org/filesupld/gender%20 health%20and%20the%20MDGs.pdf (accessed October 2005)

053 Mainstreaming gender at forum 6: a briefing document and resource guide
DOYAL, LESLEY. Geneva, Global Forum for Health Research, 2003. 60 p. ISBN 2-940286-14-0
The Global Forum for Health Research approaches gender issues with the aims of ensuring better science and to promote gender equity, and is committed to mainstreaming gender in all of its work. A plenary session at Forum 6 in Arusha, Tanzania in November 2002 focuses on progress in gender issues. Parallel sessions review gender and infectious and tropical diseases; gender, mental health and disability; gender and non-communicable diseases; violence against women; gender, sexual and reproductive health; gender, work and occupational health, and gender and child health research. The presentations demonstrate the importance of sex and gender differences in various aspects of daily life. Sensitivity to gender in health research is important to avoid wasting limited resources, and in the development of strategies to close the 10/90 gap.

http://www.globalforumhealth.org/filesupld/main streaming%20gender.pdf (accessed October 2005)

054 Sex, gender and the 10/90 gap in health research: a briefing document and resource guide
DOYAL, LESLEY. Geneva, Global Forum for Health Research, 2002. 15 p. ISBN 2-940286-08-6
The aim of the document is to provide a resource for researchers who wish to incorporate gender concerns into their work in systematic and appropriate ways. Part 1 begins with a brief

account of the arguments for gender sensitivity in health research especially in the context of poverty and social exclusion. It then goes on to explore the implications of these arguments for the research process itself. Part 2 provides a range of resources for those who wish to explore these issues further. These include articles, books and practical tools, as well as a guide to relevant websites.

http://www.globalforumhealth.org/filesupld/sex%20 gender.pdf (accessed October 2005)

055 How to integrate gender into HIV/AIDS programs: using lessons learned from USAID and partner organizations
ECKMAN, ANNE; HUNTLEY, BLAKLEY; BHUYAN, ANITA. Washington, DC, Gender and HIV/AIDS Task Force, Interagency gender Working Group (IGWG), United States Agency for International Development (USAID), 2004, 53 p.
The ability to integrate gender issues in a practical way into HIV/AIDS programmes is key for their success, and the reduction of HIV. Key gender issues and promising interventions have been identified through interviews with nearly 60 programme managers from the United States Agency for International Development (USAID) and its partners. They highlight what needs to be done to understand and address gender issues in relation to HIV/AIDS. Integrating a gender perspective increases the impact of programmes. Guidance for future programmes is provided by examining how responses may have unintentionally worsened gender inequalities, accommodated current gender norms, or sought to transform gender relationships. Cross-references to examples of promising interventions are given. Many promising interventions appear in only one programme, revealing the potential for shared best practices and systematic integration across different programmes. Gaps and emerging issues are also identified.

http://www.prb.org/pdf04/HowToIntegrGendrHIV.pdf (accessed October 2005)

056 'En-gendering' the Millennium Development Goals (MDGs) on health
Geneva, World Health Organization (WHO), 2003. 11 p.
Of the 8 Millennium Development Goals (MDGs), only no. 3 is specifically about gender, calling for the elimination of gender disparity in education. However, gender is important for all of the MDGs. The Department of Gender and Women's Health (GWH) of the World Health Organization (WHO) has therefore provided accompanying texts to the health-related MDGs 1, 4, 5, 6 and 7 to ensure that gender is addressed. In the case of Goal 1, to eradicate extreme poverty and hunger, this means examining potential inequities in nutritional, medical or other care standards. Goal 4, to reduce child mortality, requires attention to differences between mortality rates for boys and girls, providing adequate resources for pregnant women, and eliminating sex differences for immunization against measles. Goal 5, to improve maternal health, requires eliminating gender discrimination with regard to nutrition, access to health care, and education: all factors which correlate with maternal health outcomes. Goal 6, to combat HIV/AIDS, malaria and other diseases, requires special attention to the higher rates of prevalence of HIV among women, related to differences in power relations between men and women, differentiated preventive measures and care-giving roles. In the case of Goal 7, to ensure environmental sustainability, the GWH texts point out that women and children are more regularly exposed to health-damaging pollutants in the home and usually have the task of collecting household fuel and water supplies.

http://www.mdgender.net/upload/monographs/ WHO_MDGs_on_Health.pdf (accessed October 2005)

057 Ensuring women's access to safe abortion: essential strategies for achieving the Millennium Development Goals
Chapel Hill, NC, Ipas, 2005. 4 p.
The MDGs lack specific mention of human rights or reproductive and sexual health, but some are related to the right to safely terminate pregnancy. The elimination of unsafe abortion as a major, preventable cause of maternal death and illness and serious violation of human rights can help to achieve MDGs 1, 3 and 5, which relate to social and economic justice, human rights and public health. As a result of the work of women's groups and health advocates, countries are increasingly changing their abortion laws within the context of women's rights to equality and non-discrimination. South Africa recognizes women's social rights, Nepal recognizes links between the rights to inherit, divorce and safely terminate pregnancies, and Mexican programmes successfully link freedom from sexual violence and the right to end pregnancies resulting from rape. The global communication is therefore called to action to promote sexual and reproductive health, including safe abortion.

http://www.ipas.org/publications/en/MDGFLY_E05_ en.pdf (accessed October 2005)

058 Women and HIV/AIDS: confronting the crisis. A joint report
ERB-LEONCAVALLO, ANN; HOLMES, GILLIAN; JACOBS, GLORIA; URDANG, STEPHANIE; VANEK, JOANN; ZARB, MICOL. Geneva, UNAIDS, UNFPA, and UNIFEM, 2004. 64 p. refs. ISBN 0-89714-708-1
The report focuses on the UNAIDS Global Coalition on Women and AIDS Initiative to stimulate remedial action, containing an analysis of and proposal for responses to AIDS among women worldwide. Prevention and treatment, the caregiving role, education and women's rights issues are all covered in separate, in-depth chapters on comparative situations in different regions of the world. With women now accounting for nearly half of HIV-infected people worldwide, the report calls for action against gender inequality, poverty and HIV/AIDS simultaneously. Unequal education, health and property-owning opportunities lead to women having less access to protection from AIDS. Stigma and discrimination against women can limit the availability of treatment, while leaving them responsible as primary caregivers. The report offers recommendations for the promotion and protection of the human rights of women and girls, setting out existing Human Rights accords and commitments. In the concluding chapter on future steps, the report details specific actions needed to ensure protection, equal access to AIDS treatment, better education, support for caregivers and zero tolerance of violence against women.
KIT Library code Br U 04-454

059 Sex work toolkit for targeted HIV/AIDS prevention and care in sex work settings
EVANS, CATRIN. Geneva, World Health Organization (WHO), 2004
The toolkit is intended as a resource to guide the development and implementation of effective HIV interventions in diverse sex work settings. It outlines key steps and issues and provides links to many documents, manuals, reports, and research studies containing more detailed and in-depth information. Each such resource or tool has been annotated to assist readers in deciding whether it is relevant to their particular situations. The toolkit is intended for use by anyone involved in HIV prevention and care initiatives in sex work settings.
http://who.arvkit.net/sw/en/index.jsp (accessed October 2005)

060 Exploring concepts of gender and health
Ottawa, Women's Health Bureau, Health Canada, 2003. p. ISBN 0-662-34144-9
The Women's Health Strategy of Health Canada is to apply gender-based analysis (GBA) in key areas. The strategy supports gender equity in the health system, aiming to ensure equality of outcome as well as equality of opportunity. GBA is explored as a catalyst for change, in terms of its legal and global foundations and its key concepts. Consideration is given to the integration of GBA into research, policy and programme development, the research process, and policy and programme development. Case studies demonstrate its application with regard to cardiovascular disease, mental health, violence, and tobacco policy. GBA is seen as instrumental in the improvement of health outcomes and the quality of health care for people in Canada.
http://www.hs-sc.gc.ca/english/women/pdf/
exploring_concepts.pdf

061 Facing the future together: report of the United Nations Secretary-General's Task Force on Women, Girls and HIV/AIDS in Southern Africa
UN Secretary General's Task Force on Women, Girls and HIV/AIDS in Southern Africa, 2004. 55 p.
The Task Force works on six issues relating to young women and girls within a broad gender framework: the prevention of HIV/AIDS; education; violence; property and inheritance rights; caring for those living with HIV/AIDS; and access to HIV/AIDS care and treatment. The Task Force focuses on Botswana, Lesotho, Malawi, Mozambique, Namibia, South Africa, Swaziland, Zambia and Zimbabwe, as the Southern African countries most severely affected by HIV/AIDS. Country visits to ascertain people's experiences, together with literature and discussions with people working on human rights, gender and development, and HIV/AIDS provide the basis for this report and recommendations for the future. The findings show that gender inequality fuels HIV infection because many women and girls cannot negotiate safer sex or turn down unwanted sex. The findings also demonstrate that HIV/AIDS deepens and exacerbates women's poverty and inequality because it requires them to do more domestic labour as they care for the sick, the dying and the orphaned.
http://womenandaids.unaids.org/regional/docs/Report%
20of%20SG%27s%20Task%20Force.pdf (accessed October 2005)

062 Strengthening HIV/AIDS programs for women: lessons for U.S. policy from Zambia and Kenya. A report of the CSIS Task Force on HIV/AIDS

FLEISCHMAN, JANET. Washington, DC, Center for Strategic and International Studies (CSIS), 2005. 28 p.

Funding of the President's Emergency Plan for AIDS Relief (PEPFAR) began in January 2004. A field mission to Kenya and Zambia in February 2005 assesses PEPFAR implementation from a gender perspective for the purpose of appropriate adjustment and strengthening of the programme. PEPFAR is a US$15 billion global programme intended to run over five years in 15 countries. Its goals are to support treatment for 2 million people living with HIV/AIDS by 2008, to prevent 7 million new infections and to support care for 10 million infected and affected by the disease. At the point of the field mission, treatment has been provided to 155,000 people and the programme is reaching 1.2 million women with services to prevent transmission from mother to child. However, efforts must be strengthened if the 2008 goal is to be reached. PEPFAR should build on the recognition that women and girls are especially vulnerable, address key gender issues in technical areas, and implement proactive strategies. While Zambia and Kenya recognize the centrality of the gender dimension of the HIV/AIDS epidemic, programmes in these countries also demonstrate some of the constraints documented by CSIS in other countries. On the basis of examples of structural programmes in Kenya and Zambia, recommendations are offered on the guidance required in the field and among implementing partners and targeted actions needed to achieve the plan's goals.

http://www.csis.org/media/csis/pubs/strengtheninghiv-aidsprograms_(fleischman).pdf

063 Approaches to reducing maternal mortality: Oxfam and the MDGs

FRASER, ARABELLA. *Gender and Development* 13(2005)1, p. 36-43 ISSN 0277-9536

Oxfam focuses on raising national and international finance for investment in work on the Millennium Development Goals (MDGs), specifically the goal to reduce maternal mortality. This is the only goal explicitly connected to women's health, providing an opportunity to draw attention to the political, cultural and economic barriers facing women when seeking health care. Shifts in perspective now see maternal health as an end in itself, rather than only a means of population control and child welfare. While family planning reduces

the number of pregnancies, for example, it does not change risks of death from complications during pregnancy. However, at least US$ 50 billion extra a year is required if the MDG to reduce maternal mortality is to be achieved. Funding needs to be predictable and long-term, rather than one-off investments and too much focus on vertical programmes. Legal, managerial and human resource reforms should accompany financing. The aim is to finance the rebuilding of health systems to provide universal, equitable coverage in countries with high maternal mortality rates.

KIT Library shelf mark: D 3030-13(2005)1

064 Strategic advocacy and maternal mortality: moving targets and the Millennium Development Goals

FREEDMAN, LYNN. *Gender and Development* 11(2003)1, p. 97-108, refs. ISSN 0277-9536

The UN General Assembly issued a Millennium Declaration in September 2000 setting out eight goals of social and economic development, the Millennium Development Goals (MDGs). Goal 5 is to increase maternal health, reducing maternal mortality by 75%. Maternal mortality accounts for approx. 515,000 deaths each year according to 1995 estimates from WHO, UNICEF, UNFPA. The rate is dramatically different in rich and poor countries: 1 in 16 women in Africa risk death in pregnancy and childbirth compared to 1 in 5,000 in Southern Europe, for example. Women's health and rights advocates need to find effective strategies to improve the situation. Previous measures providing safe abortion services and trained traditional birth attendants are essential to health services, but do not usually prevent deaths when obstetric complications occur. Risk-screening programmes have also proved ineffective, because such complications are unpredictable. Yet 80% of maternal deaths are caused by obstetric complications that could be treated with emergency obstetric care (EmOC). Access to EmOC by all women is therefore necessary for the MDG target to be reached. A maternal mortality strategy that focuses on EmOC would also give structure to health and human rights advocacy and simultaneously provide a synergistic link to HIV, tuberculosis and other health issues.

KIT Library shelf mark: D 3030-11(2003)1

065 Who's got the power? Transforming health systems for women and children: achieving the Millennium Development Goals (MDGs)

FREEDMAN, L.P.; WALDMAN, R.J.; DE PINHO, H.; WIRTH, M.E. *Task Force on Child Health and Maternal Health UN Millennium Project.* London,

Earthscan for UNDP, 2005. 185 p. ISBN 1-84407-224-X

Governments and international agencies can take concrete steps to ensure that health interventions have significant effects on all aspects of development and the reduction of poverty. Providing an analytical context, the task force looks at global health from three perspectives, first principles of equity and human rights, the health systems crisis, and the basis for and challenges of scaling up reforms. Examination of the status of health and key interventions is broken down into links between maternal health and child health, child and adolescent health as separate categories, sexual and reproductive health, the status of health in conflict zones and among displaced populations, and maternal mortality and morbidity. In discussing the creation of a health workforce to meet the MDGs, attention is given to market-based approaches, definition, redistribution, financing, organization and management. The MDGs numbers 4: child health, neonatal mortality and nutrition and 5: improving maternal health, are considered in terms of the targets and indicators used to monitor equity and health systems, and their role in providing health information. Global policies and funding frameworks are reviewed to assess their influence, and conclusions provide the basis for further recommendations.
http://www.unmillenniumproject.org/reports/tf_health.htm (accessed October 2005)
KIT Library shelf mark: U 04-400

066 **Transforming health systems to improve the lives of women and children**
FREEDMAN, LYNN P.; WALDMAN, RONALD J.; DE PINHO, HELEN; WIRTH, MEG E.; CHOWDHURY, A. MUSHTAQUE R.; ROSENFIELD, ALLAN. Lancet 365(2005) March 12, p. 997-1000, refs. ISSN 0140-6736
What makes the Millennium Development Goals (MDGs) different from other goals for reducing mortality and increasing access to health interventions is that they are embedded in a wider poverty-reduction initiative. They have unprecedented support from governments and multilateral organizations. Of the 10.8 million children who die every year, nearly 4 million are less than 1 month old. Malnutrition is a contributing factor in more than half of all child deaths. Basic interventions exist, which are fairly simple and cost-effective, for the protection and promotion of sexual and reproductive health and rights, which would potentially reduce child deaths. Yet millions of people, predominantly in sub-Saharan Africa and Southern Asia, do not have access to them.

Health systems are a fundamental building block of an integrated poverty-reduction strategy. A fixation on short-term and short-lived successes may sidetrack human rights considerations. National governments and donors must invest in more systemic strategies for longer term, sustainable results. Substantial new investment is needed for improvement to happen. What is needed is a redistribution of power and resources between countries and within households, communities and health systems. A clear and strong moral and political commitment will be needed. as well as knowledge and money, to achieve the MDGs.
http://www.unmillenniumproject.org/documents/TheLancetChildHealthMaternalHealth.pdf (accessed October 2005)
KIT Library shelf mark: E 1927-365(2005)March 12

067 **ICPD at ten: the world reaffirms Cairo. Official outcomes of the ICPD at ten review**
FUERSICH, C.M. New York, NY, United Nations Population Fund (UNFPA), 2005. 124 p.
This publication presents a compilation of the official outcomes of the ten-year review of the International Conference on Population and Development (ICPD), which was held in Cairo, Egypt, in 1994. This collection of declarations, resolutions and agreements, adopted by regional and global inter-governmental bodies during 2002-2004, serves as a mid-point appraisal and a record of progress toward achieving the goals of the twenty-year ICPD Programme of Action and the ICPD+ 5 Key Actions for the Further Implementation of the Programme of Action of the International Conference on Population and Development.
www.unfpa.org/upload/lib_pub_file/404_filename_reaffirming_cairo.pdf (accessed October 2005)

068 **Fulfilling reproductive rights for women affected by HIV: a tool for monitoring achievement of Millennium Development Goals**
Center for Health and Gender Equity (CHANGE), International Community of Women Living with HIV/AIDS (ICW), and Pacific Institute for Women's Health (PIWH), 2005. 14 p.
On 8 March 2004, over 25 national and international organizations presented a statement to the secretariat of the UN Commission on the Status of Women that highlighted neglected areas in HIV-positive women's reproductive health. Representatives of four organizations (Ipas, the International Community of Women Living with HIV/AIDS (ICW), the Pacific Institute for Women's Health and the Center for Health and Gender Equity (CHANGE)) used that statement to develop this practical tool to help address

those areas of reproductive health: involvement of HIV-positive women in policy making and programme implementation, fertility control that meets HIV-positive women's needs, and research on antiretroviral therapy in relation to fertility. The document is organized in five sections: (1) introduces the relevant MDGs and neglected areas of reproductive health; (2) contains brief background information on the issues; (3) provides the data collection questions linked to MDGs 5 and 6; (4) gives some ideas on how the collected data can be used; and (5) lists the organizations that support use of this tool.
http://www.ipas.org/publications/en/RRHIV_E04_en.pdf (accessed October 2005)

069 Female genital mutilation (FGM), MDGs, PRSP, and the Agenda 2015: what are the linkages?
GAHN, GABI. Eschborn, Deutsche Gesellschaft für technische Zusammenarbeit (GTZ), 2004. 11 p.
The Millennium Development Goals include specific goals towards gender equality and women's empowerment, reduced child mortality and improved maternal health. This includes the right to physical integrity and reproductive health. Female genital mutilation (FGM) is a violation of human rights and an infringement of the rights of the child. FGM is closely linked to gender inequalities in the societies where it is practiced. Evidence indicates that FGM can give rise to complications during childbirth leading to stillbirth or neonatal death. It is a threat to safe motherhood, and major health complications in pregnancy, childbirth and the postpartum period are associated with it, thus it could be a contributing factor in many maternal deaths. The reduction of FGM should result in reduced maternal and child mortality rates. Poverty Reduction Strategy Papers (PRSPs) are a tool for governments of low-income countries for the development of national policies and programmes for the reduction of poverty. PRSPs are becoming the major basis for German development cooperation activities. Since the PRSPs should include the gender dimension, this would provide a platform for strategies to eliminate FGM. A gendered poverty analysis is still limited in many PRSPs, and stakeholders with the process must address the gender and human rights-related aspects of FGM, if it is to be seen as part of gender-based discrimination in general. The German government's contribution towards the 2015 Agenda is described in its Programme of Action to Combat Poverty, containing priority

areas linked with FGM, gender equality, the empowerment of women and human rights.
http://www2.gtz.de/fgm/downloads/e-FGM_MDGs_PRSP_ohneDB.pdf (accessed October 2005)

070 Participatory impact monitoring through action research: lessons from the generation dialogue and training for uncircumcised girls in Guinea
GAHN, GABI; FINKE, EMANUELA. Eschborn, Deutsche Gesellschaft für technische Zusammenarbeit (GTZ), 2005. 15 p.
Participatory monitoring is a basic means of enabling organizations to record and evaluate the impact of activities and strategies that are implemented. Programmes to abandon or prevent Female genital mutilation (FGM) must take multiple socio-cultural aspects into consideration. Those which empower women and establish dialogues with men have the best chances of achieving effective change. Two action research approaches to monitor the outcomes and impact of the work of NGOs and community members were used in Guinea: (1) the generation dialogue and (2) training for uncircumcised girls. The activities helped community members to reflect on their attitudes and practices and studies provided a useful communication tool for the target groups. The NGOs gained important information and insights for use in designing future activities. The two approaches had a measurable impact on families in the region. Partner organizations now play a new role as facilitators who initiate processes and jointly review the impact, which requires a change of attitude and new skills.
http://afronets.org/files/Impact-monitoring-en.pdf (accessed October 2005)

071 Reproductive health, gender, and development: an international perspective. A festschrift for Prof. Kuttan Mahadevan
GAO, ERSHENG (ed.). Delhi, B.R., 2003. 389 p. refs. ISBN 81-7646-328-0
Adolescent reproductive health issues are seen through studies in Guyana and Uttar Pradesh, India, to be influenced by education and home instruction about sexuality and family planning. In China, a dramatic decline in age for girls' first menstruation could be linked to year of birth, ethnicity, religion, education, socioeconomic and cultural differences. Foetal loss in India is higher among adolescents, who have had inadequate reproductive health education. Among adult women in sub-Saharan Africa, gender inequality influences reproduction decisions due to different attitudes towards contraception, which is also linked to education. In China, women's

gender and health: policy and practice

attitudes towards pre-marital sex plays an important role in pregnancy and abortion among unmarried women, and the frequency of sexual intercourse is linked to socio-graphic factors. In India, hazardous work influences women and children's morbidity profile and health problems are related to local socioeconomic conditions and relationships to doctors and healers among women in rural Tamil Nadu, India. Strategies for the control of HIV/AIDS and other sexually transmitted diseases (STDs) is studied in Uganda and among women in prostitution in Tamil Nadu, as well as the empowerment of women as an approach to the control of STDs. Finally, strategies for health planning and sustainable development are considered through study of the features of medical care, socioeconomic developments and demographic transitions in different parts of the world.

KIT Library shelf mark: P 04-2397

072 Gender analysis in health: a review of selected tools
Geneva, World Health Organization (WHO), 2002. 94 p. refs. ISBN 9-24-159040-8
The review clarifies the content of the different tools available for gender analysis and their usefulness for health issues. It assumes an understanding of the challenges of mainstreaming gender in general and of the WHO Gender Policy in particular. Different institutions have produced tools to address gender issues from different perspectives and with different objectives. Some are intended to involve both men and women equally in social and economic development programmes, and in some cases also to transform gender relations, so as to ensure the maximum effectiveness of programmes. Most aim to reduce gender inequalities. The first section of Part 1 of the review is an analysis of the tools according to gender, situation, situation, research methods, programming strategies and strategies for institutional change. The second section focuses on the impact of gender on health and health care: social determinants, behaviour, quality, promotion, financing, policy, consultation and participation. Part I concludes that most tools not only require prior skill in gender analysis, they require specific attention to gender alone in addition to the other dimensions of equity. In that sense, they may require more time that is often available to those who must address many issues in an integrated way at short notice, without the support of gender analysts. While the review raises questions about the nature and role of these tools in general, it recognizes their potential for training purposes. Part II of the review summarizes the aspects of

each tool that may be useful to WHO, describing its purpose, content, usefulness and limitations for analysis of health issues.
http://www.who.int/entity/gender/documents/en/Gender. analysis.pdf (accessed October 2005)

073 Gender and health: a technical paper
WHO/FRH/WHD/98.16. Geneva, World Health Organization (WHO), 1998
A gender analysis of health and health care issues helps to identify, analyse and redress inequalities between the sexes. Gender-sensitive policies and programmes need to be explicitly built into original objectives for this to happen. This requires preliminary data collection and analysis under consideration of the broader contextual issues. Gender roles influence the division of labour and the status assigned to men and women, which in turn has consequences for health. Three case studies examine tropical infectious diseases, HIV/AIDS and other sexually transmitted diseases, and violence and injuries. They identify both biological and social influences in health problems among women and men, concluding that women are the more disadvantaged. Gender inequalities also have an impact on health care. Evidence indicates a gender bias in medical research and inequities in access to health care and in the quality of care. If women are to be more visible, research needs to be reconfigured, providing a more accurate reflection of women's situations in health statistics. 'Gender blindness' often leads to gender being overlooked as a key determinant of social inequality. Gender concerns therefore need to be identified in the policy environment, and incorporated into health sector reform. As a result of efforts by the Women's Health & Development Programme and the Gender Working Group convened in 1996, gender equality and equity concerns were to be mainstreamed into all WHO research, policies, programmes and projects by 2002.
http://www.who.int/docstore/gender-and-health/pages/ WHO%20-%20Gender%20and%20Health%20 Technical%20Paper.htm (Ms Word 97) (accessed October 2005)
http://www.who.int/reproductive-health/publications/ WHD_98_16_gender_and_health_technical_paper/WHD_ 98_16_table_of_contents_en.html (HTML) (accessed October 2005)

074 Gender and HIV/AIDS: guidelines for integrating a gender focus into NGO work on HIV/AIDS
London, Save the Children, ActionAid, Agency for Co-operation and Research in Development (ACORD), 2002. 71 p. ISBN 1-84187-061-7

By the end of 2001, 40 million people had been infected with HIV. The World Health Organization WHO estimates around 14,000 new infections daily. The effect is devastating. Life expectancy in some regions has dropped by 25 years. Children's deaths are increasing rapidly due to mother-to-child transmission. Women and girls are more vulnerable to infection, and their vulnerability has wider social and economic effects as well as being a more than physical concern. Young people are particularly vulnerable. NGOs need to recognize links between development, gender and the spread of HIV/AIDS. These guidelines provide a framework for analysis to support staff training and awareness-raising and data collection in the community. Methodologies include the Stepping Stones method, participatory learning and appraisal (PLA) tools, tools for gender analysis and Child Rights Programming. PLAs have been implemented in Ghana for gender and sexual health, in Sri Lanka for the appraisal of sexual health needs and in Peru to support work with young people on sexual and reproductive health. The concluding part of the manual provides a resource list of useful books and documents.
KIT Library shelf mark: G 04-10

075 Gender and HIV/AIDS electronic library (on CD-ROM)
New York, NY, United Nations Development Fund for Women (UNIFEM), 2005
To promote understanding, knowledge sharing, and action on HIV/AIDS as a gender equality and human rights issue, UNIFEM with support from the Joint United Nations Programme of HIV/AIDS (UNAIDS), has developed this electronic library on CD-ROM. It is based on UNIFEM's Gender and HIV/AIDS web portal and compiles resources produced by a variety of organizations working on HIV/AIDS, including cutting-edge research and studies, training resources and tools, and multimedia advocacy materials. All information can be searched using a variety of criteria. In addition, resources are complemented by a feature called the 'e-Course Builder' that allows users to create and edit a tailored electronic course or report in HTML format, drawing from the materials contained in the CD-ROM. Topic areas are: gender mainstreaming and HIV/AIDS; gender, sexuality and power relations; gender, human rights and HIV/AIDS; prevention, treatment and care; legislation and policy; adolescents and youth; gender, HIV/AIDS, and conflict; stigma and discrimination; violence against women and HIV/AIDS; the care economy and women's unpaid work; HIV/AIDS in the workplace; men and masculinities; people living with HIV/AIDS.
To obtain a copy of the Gender and HIV/AIDS electronic library, please contact UNIFEM by e-mail at unifem@genderandaids.org

075a Gender, health, and development in the Americas: basic indicators 2005
Washington, DC, Pan American Health Organization, UNFPA and UNIFEM, 2005. 24 p.
This publication provides government, civil society, academia, and other cooperation agencies with a set of basic statistical indicators that illustrate the differences between women and men in terms of health status and its socioeconomic determinants. It includes a group of indicators that refer to conditions that exclusively or differentially affect women and men and are available in most countries. In addition to some internationally defined indicators for monitoring attainment of the MDGs, disaggregated by sex, the brochure also presents some indicators of priority gender and health issues for which information is available in only a limited number of countries.
http://www.unifem.org/attachments/products/web GENDERhlth05eng.pdf (accessed November 2005)

076 Gender inequalities and health sector reform
Policy Briefings for Health Sector Reform (2000)2. Liverpool, Liverpool School of Tropical Medicine, 2000. 4 p.
Economic and social inequalities between men and women need to be taken into consideration when policies are developed relating to health sector reform. Key elements of health sector reform often have implications for gender equity. Such elements include improvements in the functioning and cost-effectiveness of health services, health financing options, human resources management, decentralization, and working with the private sector. Brief case studies illustrate the links between health programmes and gender analysis. Gender analysis can be addressed when reforming the health sector in several ways: by improving data collection, monitoring and evaluation; by building capacity for gender analysis and action into the health system; by developing systems for improving the quality of service provision, and by the greater involvement of stakeholders in the planning and management of services.
http://www.liv.ac.uk/lstm/hsr/download/genderpb.pdf (accessed October 2005)

077 Gender mainstreaming in the health sector: experiences in Commonwealth countries
New gender mainstreaming series on development issues. London, Commonwealth Secretariat, 2002. 87 p. ISBN 0-85092-733-1
Low levels of women's health in less developed countries is a major obstacle to development. If women are to have better access to health services, they must be able to work at all levels of the health sector, together with men, to ensure attention to their specific needs. Gender equality has become a priority for action at the international level. Overviews show the evolution of approaches to women's health in the 20th century and list international landmarks in women's equality from 1949 to 1995. The achievement of gender equality necessitates an enabling environment, developed by means of a Gender Management System (GMS). A series of Commonwealth workshops has provided a consensus of the status of gender mainstreaming in Africa, Asia, the Caribbean and the South Pacific. They identified critical gaps in the enabling environment, between policy making and implementation, and between gender awareness and (changed) behaviour. Gender mainstreaming means integrating gender concerns within development policies and strategies. It also means taking a gender perspective to the existing development agenda. Examples of the detailed plans of action developed at the Commonwealth workshops include definition of a vision, and the objectives and priorities for the establishment of a GMS in health.
KIT Library shelf mark: N 03-692

078 Gender perspectives for better health and welfare systems development. Proceedings of the Fourth international Meeting on Women and Health.
WHO/WKC/SYM/04.2. Kobe, World Health Organization Center for Health Development, 2004. 140 p.
The Fourth International Meeting on Women and Health organized by the WHO Centre for Health Development (WHO Kobe Centre – WKC) was held from 5-8 October 2003 in Dar es Salaam, United Republic of Tanzania, in collaboration with the Ministry of Health of the Government of the United Republic of Tanzania, and is referred to as the Tanzania Meeting. The Tanzania Meeting follows the WKC's three International Meetings on Women and Health held since 2000. At the Third International Meeting on Women and Health in 2002 participants endorsed the Kobe Plan of Action for Women and Health (POA) and four international volunteer Task Forces

were established to implement the POA. One of the objectives of the Fourth Meeting was to report on the progress made on the implementation of the POA and to consider strategies to expand it further. Recommendations were made to guide the next phase of implementing the POA, including to formulate a core set of gender-sensitive leading health indicators; to promote the use of gender-based analysis throughout the research, policy, programme development, and knowledge transfer process, and to encourage women's leadership and empowerment.
http://www.who.or.jp/library/0310_p.pdf (accessed October 2005)

079 Gender, women and health: incorporating a gender perspective into the mainstream of WHO's policies and programmes. Report by the Secretariat
EB116/13. Geneva, World Health Organization (WHO), 2005. 4 p.
Although the United Nations Millennium Declaration and other international agreements recognize the importance of gender equity in all spheres of life, including access to health care, few significant changes have yet occurred in the health sector. Medical care and services are often inadequately attuned to the specific needs and concerns of men and women. Specific tools, guidelines and training are needed to help public health professionals to incorporate gender considerations. A global strategy and action plan, including implementation accountability mechanisms, is being prepared for submission to the governing bodies of regions and countries.
http://www.who.int/gb/ebwha/pdf_files/EB116/B116_13-en.pdf (accessed October 2005)

080 Gendered health systems biased against maternal survival: preliminary findings from Koppal, Karnataka, India
GEORGE, ASHA; IYER, ADITI; SEN, GITA. *IDS Working Paper 253*. Brighton, Institute of Development Studies (IDS), 2005. 55 p. ISBN 1-85864-880-7
The context of pregnant women's lives and the plural health systems they encounter in Koppal, a state of Karnataka, south India, is outlined. Preliminary survey findings are combined with qualitative work to illustrate the dynamics involved in seeking and receiving obstetric care. Despite high levels of poverty and scarce resources supporting primary health care in the region, women with obstetric complications do access a range of health providers. Yet they still die. Although addressing the technical and managerial capacity constraints to ensuring

annotated bibliography

equitable access to emergency obstetric care is essential, it is argued that maternal well being and survival cannot be effectively ensured without confronting the gender biases that also constrain health systems from supporting women's health and saving women's lives. These biases are analysed as failures in acknowledgement and accountability for pregnant women's needs and conclude with strategic steps to effectively respond to the situation that encompass technical, managerial and political action. (from authors' summary)
http://www.ids.ac.uk/ids/bookshop/wp/wp253.pdf (accessed October 2005)

081 The unfinished agenda for reproductive health: priorities for the next 10 years
GERMAIN, ADRIENNE; KIDWELL, J.
International Family Planning Perspectives 31(2005)2, p. 90-93 ISSN 0190-3187
Despite progress on the sexual and reproductive health and rights agenda agreed upon in Cairo, there are still many challenges ahead. Four top priorities to address the unfinished reproductive health agenda are: reproductive health and the Millennium Development Goals; the feminization of the HIV/AIDS epidemic; comprehensive sex education; and prevention of unsafe abortion.
http://www.agi-usa.org/pubs/journals/3109005.pdf (accessed October 2005)
KIT Library shelf mark: H 1795-31(2005)2

082 Sex and the hemisphere: the Millennium Development Goals and sexual and reproductive health in Latin America and the Caribbean. A report on two symposia: New York, 20 October 2004, and Rio de Janeiro, 30 November 2004
GIRARD, FRANCOISE. London, International Planned Parenthood Federation/Western Hemisphere Region (IPPF/WHR), 2004. 50 p.
Realizing the Millennium Development Goals (MDGs) and eradicating poverty requires implementation of sexual and reproductive health and rights programmes. The greatest challenge in Latin America and the Caribbean is inequality, and existing policies must be challenged for its lack of concern about the well being of populations. The privatization of health systems has had a negative impact on the poorest, particularly women. Although sexual and reproductive health services, including HIV treatment, would be costly, they would result in important health and economic benefits. It is important to consider these issues within a broad social justice context. Activism is essential to policy change, and all social justice movements should be enlisted and mobilized. NGOs and governments can push for improved targets.

Women's organizations can build alliances with family-planning associations and others. Doctors and health personnel can join activists in pushing for renewed implementation of sexual and reproductive health agreements according to the ICPD Programme of Action, the Beijing Platform for Action and the UN Millennium Project report. Without civil society there would have been no past achievements, and future hurdles would be insurmountable.
http://www.ippfwhr.org/publications/download/mono raphs/Symposia_Report.pdf (accessed October 2005)

083 Girls, HIV/AIDS and education
New York, NY, United Nations Children's Fund (UNICEF), 2004. 39 p.
Providing good-quality basic education and skills-based prevention education is fundamental to reversing the spread of HIV/AIDS, particularly for girls. Girls are at greater risk of contracting the disease, bear a disproportionate share of its burden and comprise the majority of new infections globally. Yet, because of persistent gender disparity, they are often denied an education and thus protection against infection. This joint project with the Global Coalition on Women and AIDS, provides graphic and tabular evidence that links sexual knowledge/behaviour and educational level among young people. It outlines three priorities that support schools in protecting girls and mitigating the impact of HIV/AIDS: (1) getting and keeping girls in school; (2) proving life skills-based education; and (3) protecting girls from gender-based school violence.
http://www.unicef.org/publications/files/Girls_HIV_ AIDS_and_Education_(English)_rev.pdf (accessed October 2005)

084 Globalization, health sector reform, gender and reproductive health
New York, NY, Reproductive Health Affinity Group (RHAG), Ford Foundation, 2004. 85 p.
Papers commissioned by the Ford Foundation Reproductive Health Affinity Group (RHAG) explore changes in economic and social policies that affect women's reproductive health and rights. Under the heading of 'Understanding the Links', Barbara Evers and Mercedes Juarez discuss a gender approach to globalization and health sector reform (HSR) and the reproductive health agenda in the context of HSR. Further papers providing experts' perspectives on the subject discuss the economic justice implications (Rosalind Petchesky), human rights implications (Rebecca Cook), the rhetoric and reality of health reforms (Priya Nanda) and key areas for strategic advocacy and citizen participation

(Vimala Ramachandran). Action points are offered for the Ford Foundation, its partners, and other interested parties.
http://www.fordfound.org/elibrary/documents/5004/toc.cfm (accessed October 2005)

085 Participation in sexual and reproductive well-being and rights
GORDON, GILL; CORNWALL, ANDREA. *Participatory Learning and Action* (2004)5, p. 73-80 ISSN 1357-938X
New challenges continue to arise in changing environments. Key issues in work on sexual and reproductive health and rights (SRHR) are: participatory HIV prevention and care work in times of crisis; links between sexuality, poverty and development, participation in connection with sexuality and gender, and the forces at work behind the agenda in participatory planning. Used sensitively, participatory approaches are a powerful tool. However, they must receive appropriate follow-up and support for them to realize SRHR and avoid retrogression and even reinforcement of power structures that threaten people's well being, and could even endanger their lives.
KIT Library shelf mark: D 3162-(2004)50

086 Beneath the surface: Regional workshop on working on gender, sexuality and HIV/AIDS in Southern Africa: questions, lessons, directions, Lusaka, Zambia, December 2-6, 2003
GREIG, ALAN. Brighton, International HIV/AIDS Alliance, 2003. 36 p.
Social norms affect the ability of men and women to protect themselves against HIV/AIDS and to cope with its impact. Women's access to sexual health knowledge and services is often limited. Social pressures on men to prove their masculinity, together with lack of understanding of sexual health issues, make them also vulnerable. This Alliance workshop to address gender and sexuality issues brought together participants from organizations in South Africa, Botswana, Zimbabwe, Namibia and Uganda. The process themes in the workshop cover targeting, accessing and engaging with community members; methods, including participatory approaches and the integration of gender and sexuality issues into existing programmes; and evaluation and sustainability. Content themes are socialization; pleasure and danger; and power and violence. An emerging issue concerns the challenge of working with men to change gender inequality.
http://www.preventgbvafrica.org/images/publications/reports/wkshprepgreigmar03.pdf (accessed October 2005)

087 Taking action to improve women's health through gender equality and women's empowerment
GROWN, CAREN; GUPTA, GEETA RAO; PANDE, ROHINI. *Lancet* 365(2005)9469, p. 541-543 ISSN 0140-6736
Despite great progress in improving women's health in recent decades, over half a million women annually die in pregnancy and childbirth due to preventable reasons, and 50% of all adults with HIV/AIDS are women. Research shows that education for girls is an important factor for improved health, reduced gender inequality, and greater empowerment for women. While universal primary education results in positive outcomes, secondary education has stronger effects. Female secondary education is associated with higher age at marriage, low fertility and mortality, good maternal care and reduced vulnerability to HIV/AIDS. Studies show that secondary schooling positively affects women's use of prenatal and delivery services and postnatal care. Sometimes, e.g. in Egypt, women with secondary education were found to be four times more likely to oppose female genital cutting than women who had never completed primary school. And secondary education can be crucial in reducing violence against women, thus positively affecting levels of unwanted pregnancies and sexually transmitted infections (including HIV/AIDS). Other important contributors to improved health for women are better transportation, water and sanitation services, better access to schooling and improved education through curriculum reform and teacher training, and the institution of women's rights to own and inherit property.
KIT Library shelf mark: E 1927-365(2005)9469

088 Addressing gender-based violence from the reproductive health/HIV sector: a literature review and analysis
GUEDES, ALESSANDRA. Washington, DC, Population Technical Assistance Project, 2004. 115 p.
At least one in every three women worldwide has been beaten, coerced into sex or otherwise abused in her lifetime. There can be many negative consequences for women's health. Gender-based violence can affect children and detract from the economic well being of societies. It is also linked to HIV/AIDS. This literature review includes programmes for both adults and adolescents, and programmes that involve men. Two elements are key in understanding gender-based violence. Firstly, the continuum of behaviours from threat and unwanted touch to rape. Secondly, the lack of

options available to women who experience such violence that do not have severe physical or social consequences. The present challenge consists of finding the most effective interventions to address gender-based violence. Given a lack of rigorous evaluation data, best practices have not yet been established. The review therefore is not an exhaustive range of approaches. Four approaches are highlighted: behaviour change communication, community mobilization, service provision, and policy. Two sections are organized around the targeted audiences of young people and refugees, internally displaced populations, and returnees.

http://www.prb.org/pdf04/AddressGendrBasedViolence. pdf (accessed October 2005)

089 Guidelines for the analysis of gender and health

Liverpool, Gender and Health Group, Liverpool School of Tropical Medicine, 1998
Guidelines are needed for gender analysis in health in order to reduce inequities and to increase the efficiency and effectiveness of health care services. The guidelines include background information, a gender analysis framework, guidance on gender-sensitive planning and outlines of possible strategies to address gender inequalities. Case studies offer examples of gender analysis in projects in India, Uganda and Zambia. Suggestions are offered as to how the guidelines can be used in various ways by different groups.

http://www.liv.ac.uk/lstm/hsr/GG-1.html (accessed October 2005)

090 Responding to Cairo: case studies of changing practice in reproductive health and family planning

HABERLAND, NICOLE; MEASHAM, DIANA (eds). New York, NY, Population Council, 2002. 462 p. ISBN 0-87834-106-4
Since the International Conference on Population and Development (ICDP) in Cairo, September 1994, the translation of the Programme of Action into effective reproductive health services has presented a major challenge. One concern is that many health interventions are small-scale, and infrequently replicated at a national level. This will require changes in national policy and strategies and the implementation of community programmes which will take far more resources and years of further work. However, policies and programmes in the last 40 years have gradually shown greater sensitivity to women's needs and improved quality of care. Persistence is still necessary if the breakthrough in reproductive health and rights introduced by the Cairo

conference is to become a widespread practical reality. The geographic and programmatic content of the case studies ranges from national policy and programme changes in China and India to community-based projects in Peru, from post-abortion care to service delivery and changing gender power norms. They provide practical information on both successes and failures.

091 Adolescent and youth reproductive health in the Asia and Near East region: status, issues, policies, and programs

HARDEE, KAREN; PINE, PAMELA; WASSON, LAUREN TAGGART. POLICY *Occasional Paper 9*. Washington, DC, POLICY Project, 2004
This synthesis presents the findings of a 13-country study of issues, policies and programmes in Bangladesh, Cambodia, Egypt, India, Indonesia, Jordan, Morocco, Nepal, Pakistan, Philippines, Sri Lanka, Vietnam and Yemen on behalf of the Asia/Near East Bureau of the United States Agency for International Development (USAID). The purpose of the assessments was to examine the reproductive health situation of young people in each country. While social and cultural contexts vary considerably among the countries, several universal challenges were observed. These included scanty research and data on the age group, lacking attention to gender inequality, insufficient information and services for young people, and inadequate policies on reproductive health among the young. The report offers recommendations to address these challenges. They include the involvement of young people in developing relevant policies and programmes, informing policy makers of their needs, educating various groups with a view to changing public opinion about the importance of these issues, promoting communication in families and gender equity in all youth-related policies and programmes, increasing access to information and services and developing further appropriate programmes.

092 Health research for the Millennium Development Goals: a report on Forum 8, Mexico City, 16-20 November 2004

STEARNS, BEVERLY PETERSON. Geneva, Global Forum for Health Research, 2005. 64 p. ISBN 2-940286-31-0
According to some assessments, the world will not achieve the MDGs by 2015. There is a need for more political commitment, a wide interpretation of the health agenda underlying

gender and health: policy and practice

specific MDG targets, more application of existing knowledge and more health research. The vicious circle of poverty and ill health will not be broken without intensified effort to close the '10/90' gap: the estimate that less of 10% of global health research resources are applied to 90% of the world's health problems. Health research is required to develop new knowledge and new technologies, especially in the areas of child and maternal health, and sexual and reproductive health. In addition, health systems need to gain access to the knowledge and technology already available, and apply them. More attention must be given to the issues of poverty and equity, to the needs of the aged and the very young, and to disadvantaged groups such as migrants, refugees and those exposed to violent conflict.

http://www.globalforumhealth.org/filesupld/publications /F8_synthesis_report.pdf (accessed October 2005)

093 Advancing reproductive health as a human right: progress toward safe abortion care in selected Asian countries since ICPD
HESSINI, LEILA. Chapel Hill, NC, Ipas, 2004. 58 p. ISBN 1-882220-76-5
Globally, women average one abortion during their reproductive years, making abortion one of the most common medical procedures in the world. Close to half of all abortions are performed under unsafe conditions, and nearly 70,000 women die annually as a result. Despite government commitments following the International Conference on Population and Development (ICDP), an estimated 34,000 deaths per year occur from unsafe abortion in Asia. Examples from India, Indonesia, Malaysia, Nepal, the Philippines and Thailand illustrate the diversity of experience related to abortion and reproductive health issues throughout the region. Political, economic, medical, social and cultural circumstances make implementation of abortion-care recommendations difficult. In spite of the many national and regional initiatives and activities that have been launched, much remains to be done. Interviews with key stakeholders in the six countries provide qualitative data, which is supplemented with data and statistics.

http://www.ipas.org/publications/en/ICPD_04/ASICPD_ E03_en.pdf (accessed October 2005)

094 HIV prevention in maternal health services: training guide
New York, NY, United Nations Population Fund (UNFPA) and EngenderHealth, 2004, 127 p. ISBN 0-89714-693-X
This training guide has been designed using participatory training approaches, which means that the exercises require the active involvement of all participants. The role of the facilitator is to guide the participants through learning activities rather than to lecture or just provide information to a passive audience. Participatory methods, such as brainstorming or role-play exercises, have been shown to be a critical feature of successful adult learning. The training guide has been developed for use by skilled, experienced trainers who are familiar with the content and objectives of each exercise. While the training guide contains information to help trainers understand each exercise, it is assumed that the trainers knows about adult learning concepts, employs a variety of training methods and techniques, and knows how to adapt materials to meet participants' need. The training guide consists of a detailed curriculum with session guides, and a series of appendices containing additional materials. The goal of the training is to build the capacity of programme managers and staff to address pregnant and postpartum clients' HIV and STI needs by offering integrated HIV and STI services within their own particular service delivery setting.

http://www.engenderhealth.org/res/offc/hiv/prevention/ pdf/hiv_prev_training_gde.pdf (accessed October 2005)

095 The HIV/Gender Continuum: how gender-sensitive are your HIV and family planning services?
New York, NY, International Planned Parenthood Federation Western Hemisphere Region (IPPF/WHR), 2002, 6 p.
The HIV/Gender Continuum is a tool to investigate how responsive an organization's services and programmes are to gender issues related to HIV prevention within an overall rights-based approach to sexual and reproductive health. Which components of your programmes and services are not gender sensitive? Somewhat gender-sensitive? Ideal? Programmes that fall to the left of the Continuum are ripe for a substantial overhaul that might require external facilitation. Programmes that fall in the middle are moving in the gender-sensitive direction and would benefit from an internal commitment to continue growth in this direction. Programmes that fall to the right are model programmes and may be able to produce best practices documents or otherwise share their experiences in this area.

http://www.ippfwhr.org/publications/download/mono graphs/gender_continuum.pdf (accessed October 2005)

annotated bibliography

137

096 Gender, equity, and indigenous women's health in the Americas
HUGHES, JESSICA. Washington, DC, Pan-American Health Organization (PAHO), 2004. 31 p. refs.
The health status, gender roles and relations of indigenous women in Canada, Ecuador, Guatemala, Mexico, Nicaragua, Peru and the United States are explored in relation to health outcomes. The specific factors of a triple burden of labour, absence of sufficient appropriate health services, national socioeconomic conditions, social instability and employment in the informal sector are seen to have severe health consequences. The latter are examined in relation to a growing incidence of HIV/AIDS, high maternal mortality rates, substance abuse, disproportionate rates of suicide and violence and higher risk of a number of diseases among women.
http://www.paho.org/English/AD/GE/IndigenousWomen-Hughes0904.pdf (accessed October 2005)

097 Gender, leprosy and leprosy control: a case study in Aceh, Indonesia
IDAWANI, CUT.; YULIZAR, M., LEVER, P., & VARKEVISSER, C.M. Amsterdam, Royal Tropical Institute (KIT), 2002. 96 p. ISBN 90-6832-717-8
In Aceh, the male/female ratio among leprosy patients appears to be stable at 1.5. Women are also less seriously affected than men although there is no significant gender difference in deformity. Differences, also for multibacillary (MB) leprosy were most pronounced in women of reproductive age. The difference was, however, insufficient to confirm the possibility of hormonal protection in women of reproductive age. Both men and women are equally late in reporting for treatment. It is important to win the trust of traditional healers, in light of strong traditional perceptions. Fear of leprosy in the community often leads to stigmatization. Stigma does not appear to be related to gender in Aceh, which is a matrilineal society, but is sometimes linked to low socio-economic status and personal characteristics. Health centres are under-utilized, and people are largely unaware that leprosy is treatable and that Multi Drug Therapy is effective and free of charge. Male leprosy workers in the community may feel inhibited in carrying out clinical examinations of young women and patients of higher rank. Case detection and diagnosis are more problematic than case holding. Once they start treatment, it is completed by almost 90% of patients.
KIT Library shelf mark: N 03-498; N 03-499

098 Implementing ICPD: what's happening in countries
BERER, MARGE. *Reproductive Health Matters* (2005)25, special issue
This collection of papers from around the world reflects on developments at country level since the International Conference on Population and Development (ICDP) in Cairo in 1994. Brazil and Argentina have started to set up services and foster public awareness of women's health policies. In Norway, it is observed that some issues that are treated as important in Norway, are neglected in donor funding policies. In the Arab countries, the patriarchal system is being challenged by better education and the improving economic situation of young women. A theme-based review looks at an emerging global movement to support women's right to safe abortion, which as progressed considerably in the last ten years. Socioeconomic factors for the achievement of reproductive health are considered in relation to women in Lebanon. Equal educational opportunities for girls are considered as an important prerequisite for the achievement of development goals. The consequences of failing AIDS policy in Africa is the subject of a speech on the vulnerability of children, and the importance of long-term provision of comprehensive reproductive care and treatment is considered in relation to HIV. There are many signs of progress, and countries are now giving more attention to issues of sexual and reproductive health. Overall, however, it appears that the gap between rich and poor, those with power and those without, is widening.
KIT Library shelf mark: D 3099-(2005)25

099 Information, education and communication: lessons from the past. Perspectives for the future
Occasional paper. Geneva, World Health Organization (WHO), 2001. 41 p. refs
An occasional paper on the lessons learned from over 20 years of information, education and communication (IEC) public health interventions for the purpose of improved reproductive health programmes and service delivery. Aside from general lessons learned as to the effectiveness and implementation of IEC, concise descriptions cover strategy planning, implementation, monitoring and evaluation, and training. Specific lessons learned with regard to reproductive health cover peer education, support groups, counselling and interpersonal communication, gender considerations, youth issues, negotiation and life skills, interactions with religious institutions, and partnerships for the integration of IEC. The paper enumerates fundamental issues to be addressed by IEC specialists and

other experts in the future, such as the increasing importance of the communication strategy. Partnerships are recognized as key for sustainable outcomes. Understanding of overall socio-cultural and political environments is paramount for appropriate IEC programmes. A coherent system must take divergent perspectives and needs into consideration, and the task of pursuing long-term IEC goals remains an evolving one requiring flexibility and forward-thinking.

http://www.who.int/reproductive-health/publications/ RHR_01_22/information_education_communication_ lessons_from_past.pdf (accessed October 2005)

100 Information on female genital cutting: what is out there? What is needed? An assessment
Washington, DC, Female Genital Cutting Interagency Working Group of the United States Agency for International Development (USAID), 2004. 21 p.

Available information and information gaps have been assessed by the Population Reference Bureau, Family Health International, PATH, the Population Council and The Manoff Group. Information was gathered by means of in-country questionnaires (186), a Survey Monkey (an Internet survey tool used by PRB), of NGOs, government agencies, research institutes and others, and a website review of 29 websites and databases. Survey Monkey respondents stated they got their information on FGC from printed materials from research or advocacy groups (83%), followed by web searches (69%) symposiums, conferences or workshops (62%), face-to-face (59%), libraries (43%) or listservs (34%). In-country respondents from eight countries declared their most important source as face-to-face communications. Access varies between countries and respondents, but in general, print materials are preferred to electronic materials. An assessment of the gaps in information shows the most needed information among Survey Monkey respondents to be best practices/evaluation results, advocacy tools and statistical information, followed by training manuals and case studies. In-country findings were generally consistent with these findings. The best available websites were found to be: Intact Network, Reproductive Health Gateway and the GTZ (Deutsche Gesellschaft für Technische Zusammenarbeit). Recommendations proposed by the collaborating agencies conducting the assessment include: better dissemination of information, information collation on operations research, sharing best practices, organizing face-to-face information exchanges, producing a policy information brief, and improving websites and information dissemination.

http://www2.gtz.de/fgm/downloads/PRB_InfoOnFGC.pdf (accessed October 2005)

101 Integrating gender into HIV/AIDS programmes: a review paper
Geneva, World Health Organization (WHO), 2003. 56 p. ISBN 92 4 159039 4

Knowledge of gender-related factors that determine vulnerability to and treatment of HIV/AIDS has increased considerably, yet implementing action based on that knowledge is difficult. Programme managers need guidelines to help them integrate gender issues, because of the greater effectiveness of HIV/AIDS programmes that acknowledge their impact. Programmes world-wide use different approaches, providing important lessons. Approaches range from those that merely 'do no harm', to 'gender sensitive' programmes to 'transformative' interventions. Ultimately, structural interventions go beyond health systems to reduce gender inequalities by empowering women and girls. The success of integration of gender concerns depends on how structural constraints and barriers are addressed. Political will and leadership must be fostered and developed at the level of state institutions to create the requisite policy environment. Initiatives should be based on equity and efficiency rationales; human rights and justice, and the recognition that gender integration results in more sustainable long-term results. That HIV/AIDS is more than a health issue, is key in addressing it. The countries most successful in reducing new infections (e.g. Senegal, Thailand and Uganda) are those using a multi-sectoral approach. Continual adaptation and gender-sensitive programming are required to meet women's and men's gender and age-specific needs within specific social and cultural contexts. In the long term, however, additional transformative and empowering programmes are essential if underlying factors contributing to the epidemic are to be eliminated.

http://whqlibdoc.who.int/publications/2003/9241590394. pdf (accessed October 2005)

102 Integrating poverty and gender into health programmes: a sourcebook for health professionals. Module on gender-based violence
Geneva, World Health Organization (WHO), 2005. 77 p. ISBN 92-9061-194-4

It is estimated that about 70% of the world's poor are women. Similarly, in the Western Pacific Region, poverty often wears a woman's face. Indicators of human poverty, including health

annotated bibliography

139

indicators, often reflect severe gender-based disparities. In this way, gender inequality is a significant determinant of health outcomes in the Region, with women and girls often at a severe societal disadvantage. Although poverty and gender significantly influence health and socioeconomic development, health professionals are not always adequately prepared to address such issues in their work. This publication aims to improve the awareness, knowledge and skills of health professionals in the Region on poverty and gender concerns. The set of modules that comprise this sourcebook are intended for use in pre-service and in-service training of health professionals. It is expected that this publication will also be of use to health policy makers and programme managers, either as a reference document or in conjunction with in-service training. All modules in the series are linked, but each one can be used on a stand-alone basis if required. There are two foundational modules that set out the conceptual framework for the analysis of poverty and gender issues in health. Each of the other modules is intended for use in conjunction with these two foundational modules. The Sourcebook also contains a module on curricular integration to support health professional educational institutions in the process of integration of poverty and gender concerns into existing curricula.

http://www.wpro.who.int/NR/rdonlyres/E517AAA7-E80B-4236-92A1-6EF28A6122B3/0/Integrating_poverty_gender_sourcebook.pdf

103 Into good hands: progress reports from the field
New York, NY, United Nations Population Fund (UNFPA), 2004. 24 p.
The 1994 UN International Conference on Population and Development in Cairo marked a shift towards a broader and rights-based definition of reproductive health. Its goal is universally accessible reproductive health care services through primary health care by 2015. While there are indications of progress in reproductive health education, access to contraception, infant mortality and skilled care during childbirth, however, the Cairo Programme of Action is still far from being implemented. It is undermined by macroeconomic factors, an increasingly conservative environment and the predominance of World Bank policies. The Millennium Development Goals position women's and children's right to health within a biological framework. U.S. funding is withheld from NGOs which promote or provide referrals for abortion.
http://www.unfpa.org/upload/lib_pub_file/378_filename_hands_en.pdf (accessed October 2005)

104 Investing in people: national progress in implementing the ICPD Programme of Action 1994-2004
New York, NY, United Nations Population Fund (UNFPA), 2004. 147 p.
At the 1994 International Conference on Population and Development (ICPD), 179 countries adopted a 20-year Programme of Action. Ten years on, national progress is clearly visible. There is confirmation that countries are adopting an incremental approach, focusing first on priorities. The formal adoption of policies, legislation, strategies and programmes demonstrates an increase in ways of addressing population, gender and reproductive health issues. There are efforts to integrate family planning services into reproductive health. A trend towards safe motherhood shows greater emphasis on attended delivery and referrals in emergency. Members of civil society, especially women's groups, are increasing involved in policy making and programming. Progress is not uniform across countries or programme areas. Attainment is being to be recognized as critical to achieving the Millennium Development Goals, with the potential for an integrated approach. Investing in people is the key to sustained economic growth, better reproductive health and rights, and population stabilization. It is possible to fulfil the promise of the ICPD.
http://www.unfpa.org/upload/lib_pub_file/284_filename_globalsurvey.pdf (accessed October 2005)

105 Involving men to address gender inequities: three case studies
Washington, DC, Inter-Agency Gender Working Group (IGWG), U.S. Agency for International Development (USAID), 2003. 70 p.
Case studies of programmes in Mexico, India and Uganda show how working with men can reduce gender-based violence, improve men's support for women's reproductive health and help prevent the transmission of HIV. The programmes demonstrate how men's assumption of their right to greater power than women is challenged. An attempt is made to demonstrate that the exercise of traditional masculine roles often has negative consequences for men as well as their partners. All three programmes evolved out of work on health, violence and related issues. They rely on a logical sequence of ideas and activities, with interactive self-discovery as a fundamental element. Facilitators recognize that they must face and resolve the same challenges as participants, thus reducing the social distance between them.
http://www.prb.org/pdf/InvolvMenToAddressGendr.pdf (accessed October 2005)

106 Positively informed: lessons plans and guidance for sexuality educators and advocates
IRVIN, ANDREA. New York, NY, International Women's Health Coalition, 2004. 196 p.
A selection of lessons and activities are provided for use in the classroom by teachers, by NGO staff members, or by country-level Ministries of Health or Education. The lesson plans are intended for 10-19 year-olds. The materials are ideas and examples that will inspire teachers and programme developers to create and publish their own materials. Following an introduction to human sexuality, the contents range from gender and sexual rights through anatomy, reproduction, sexual orientation, relationships, behaviour, decision making, STIs and HIV/AIDS, contraception, unintended pregnancy and abortion, and sexual violence and harmful practices. Recommendations and guidance are offered on guiding principles, life behaviours, getting community support, designing courses and becoming a sexuality educator.
http://www.iwhc.org/resources/positivelyinformed/index.cfm (accessed October 2005)

107 It takes 2: partnering with men in sexual and reproductive health
New York, NY, United Nations Population Fund (UNFPA), 2003. 59 p. ISBN 0-89714-656-5
It is important to work with men, as well as women, to improve reproductive health. UNFPA provides information and guidance on adopting a socio-cultural perspective and integrating gender in programmes. Use of a selection of strategies and indicators for successful implementation, monitoring and evaluation are practical aids for the design and evaluation of new projects.
http://www.unfpa.org/upload/lib_pub_file/153_filename_ItTakes2.pdf (accessed October 2005)

108 Restructuring the health system: experience of advocates for gender equity in Bangladesh
JAHAN, ROUNAQ. *Reproductive Health Matters* (2003)21, p. 183-191 ISSN 0968-8080
An analysis of health sector reforms and reform advocates in Bangladesh from 1995 to 2002 is presented. The focus is on the gaps between reform design by advocates and implementation through government/donor-driver programmes. Advocacy has succeeded in heightening awareness of social and gender inequality and increasing the involvement of women in reform design. However, a government change in 2001 is linked to a weakening of the capacity to implement the reforms, due to a shift in focus and priorities. Successful continuation of the implementation of reforms is seen to depend on sustained civil society advocacy and alliances with other groups such as the women's movement, in addition to promotion through government channels.
KIT Library code D 3099-(2003)21

109 Female genital cutting among the Somali of Kenya and management of its complications
JALDESA, GUYO W.; ASKEW, IAN; NJUE, CAROLYNE; WANJIRU, MONICA. New York, NY, Population Council, 2005. 34 p.
Infibulation (type III or Pharaonic circumcision), a severe form of female genital cutting (FGC), is widely practiced among the Somali women in the North Eastern Province of Kenya for reasons of religion, family honour, and to ensure virginity until marriage. FGC is not seen by this group as a rite of passage. The health sector is not equipped to serve women who have been cut, particularly pregnant infibulated women. Safe motherhood services in general are not easily accessible in the Province. There is evidence that perinatal complications occur 2-3 times more frequently among Somali women than among women originating from other countries. Maternal mortality in the surveyed group is also many times higher than in other provinces. While there are arguments indicating that FGC is not an Islamic requirement, it is difficult to dispute a belief that it is Sunna, i.e., recommended by the Prophet Mohamed. Nevertheless, arguments relating to religious teachings and sexuality are more likely to prove effective in bringing about change in behaviour in this group than reference to illegality or infringement of internationally-defined human rights. A case can be made for replacing infibulation with less severe FGC types I or II.
http://www.popcouncil.org/pdfs/frontiers/FR_Final Reports/Kenya_Somali.pdf (accessed October 2005)

110 Female sex worker HIV prevention projects: lessons learnt from Papua New Guinea, India and Bangladesh
JENKINS, CAROL. *UNAIDS Case Study.*
UNAIDS Best Practice Collection. Geneva, UNAIDS, 2000. 130 p. ISBN 92-9173-014-9
Projects in widely varying sets of circumstances illustrate aspects of good practices in sex worker interventions, and also provide lessons as to why some actions fail. Rising numbers of HIV infections has led to many countries focusing on female sex workers as being dangerous agents of infection, and their clients as unwitting victims. But from another perspective, sex workers are themselves highly vulnerable to infection. Enabling approaches to remove social restraints on safer sex or put barriers in the way of unsafe sex demonstrate more successful results. The

Transex project in Papua New Guinea studies sex and transport workers, police and security men. The Sonagachi project in India focuses on a red light district in Calcutta, and the Shakti project in Bangladesh refers to brothels and street-based sex workers. The Transex and Sonagachi projects address social and sexual norms with the objective of bringing about changes in behaviour, while the Shakti project works to improve condom usage, without confronting power structures. One major lesson learned is that protecting the human rights of sex workers is one of the best ways of protecting other societal groups from HIV infection.
http://www.unaids.org/NetTools/Misc/DocInfo.aspx? href=http://gva-doc-owl/WEBcontent/Documents/pub/ Publications/IRC-pub05/JC438-FemSexWork_en.pdf (accessed October 2005)

111 Empowering women and girls: challenges and strategies in gender equality. Partnership report
KAHURANANGA, RUTH; MAFANI, MARINA. Monrovia, CA, World Vision International, 2005. 101 p.
Eight case studies and articles written by experts in Kenya, Burundi, Afghanistan, Brazil, Nicaragua, Romania, Mongolia and India describe the challenges, achievements and gaps experienced in the empowerment of women and girls in their countries. Each article contains specific recommendations for addressing specific issues, from violence against women and girls, girl child exploitation, trafficking, child labour, abuse and neglect, to HIV/AIDS among women, maternal health, and the disproportionate suffering of women in armed conflict zones. The recommendations constitute a briefing paper for national governments presenting to the UN on the progress made in implementing the Beijing Platform for Action, at the 49th Session of the UN Commission on the Status of Women, 28 February – 11 March 2005. The Millennium Development Goals (MDGs) established at the UN Millennium Summit 2000 deal with poverty and hunger, universal primary education, child mortality, material health, HIV/AIDS, malaria and other diseases, environmental sustainability and global partnerships. While Goal 3 deals specifically with promoting gender equality and empowering women, all 8 MDGs show significant overlaps with the 12 critical areas of the Beijing Platform of Action resulting from the Fourth World Congress on Women in Beijing (1995). Since the issues addressed by the MDGs affect women and girls disproportionately, all MDGs therefore need to incorporate a gender perspective.
http://www.child-rights.org/PolicyAdvocacy/pahome2. 5.nsf/allreports/48DFE2BBABABCDED88256F8E001B3E CE/$file/CSW05rev.pdf (accessed October 2005)

112 Integrating SRH and HIV/AIDS services: Pathfinder International's experience synergizing health initiatives
KANE, MARGOT M.; COLTON, TAYLA C. Watertown, MA, Pathfinder International, 2005. 16 p.
A description of the need for and provision of USAID and privately-financed, integrated family planning, sexual and reproductive health (SRH) and HIV/AIDS services by the Pathfinder International organization, detailing the relative advantages and disadvantages. Integrated services more effectively combat AIDS by reaching more people otherwise handled separately, although there is a need for training, supplies and logistics for both sets of services. Pathfinder integration strategies support the focus on women as increasingly vulnerable to HIV/AIDS. Services are provided through clinics and community-based provider networks in India and Brazil as well as several African countries. Pathfinder was one of the first international organizations to use private funds to support family planning activities in Ethiopia, and continues to deliver USAID-funded, integrated services there. It is expanding its community-based services in cooperation with other international agencies and local NGOs. Local partners are supported in programmes to provide SRH services for young people in several African countries. Integrated service projects also target vulnerable groups otherwise often stigmatized and discouraged from seeking services. Interventions with sex workers and their clients are implemented in Asia, Africa and South America. The document concludes with a summary of the lessons learned on integration as well as a list of challenges reflecting the oversight and under-funding of integrated initiatives both globally and locally.
http://www.pathfind.org/site/DocServer/FP_HIV_ Integration_web_copy.pdf?docID=3461 (accessed October 2005)

113 The gender dimensions of HIV/AIDS challenges for South Asia: extracts from a regional scan and South Asian Regional Consultation
KHANNA, AKSHAY; DHAR, SUNEETA. Geneva, Joint United Nations Programme on HIV/AIDS (UNAIDS), 2004. 42 p. ISBN 92-9173-396-2

The interrelationship of gender and HIV/AIDS in the South Asian context is analysed. A regional rapid scan involving seven countries of the region culminated in the Regional Consultation on Gender and HIV/AIDS jointly convened in May 2004 by UNIFEM Regional Office and UNAIDS South Asia Inter-country Team. The paper presents an overview of the legal and policy framework and the status of women, describes some initiatives launched in the region on relationship between gender and HIV/AIDS and finally comes up with a set of recommendations for future action.
http://www.synergyaids.com/documents/SEAsia_Gender Dimensions.pdf (accessed October 2005)

114 Mainstreaming gender into HIV/AIDS action: priorities for interventions focusing on women and girls
KOITELEL, PHILIP OLE. AZTRAMADE (Agency for Strategic Management & Development) Consulting, 2004. 8 p.
Guidelines for the integration of gender concerns into the Kenya national HIV/AIDS Strategic Plan propose analysis and strategies based on field studies in 2001-2002 and published UNAIDS best practices. Men, and especially young boys, are vulnerable to HIV/AIDS in societies that celebrate promiscuity, without adequate understanding of sexual health issues. The risks are increased by their higher susceptibility to substance abuse and family disruption through mobility for work or military service. Prioritizing interventions for women and girls is, however, proposed because the rate of incidence is faster and age at infection is earlier among women than among men. Findings show that socially-constructed male and female roles influence men's and women's, girls' and boys' ability to protect themselves or handle the impact of HIV/AIDS. Gender-related factors influence the extent of their vulnerability, the ways they are affected and what responses are open to them in different communities. Since the spread of HIV/AIDS in Africa is fuelled by gender inequalities, therefore, effective prevention and control of its impact requires recognition of women's rights and the empowerment of women as an important tool in the fight against the disease.
http://www.gdnet.org/fulltext/koitelel.pdf (accessed October 2005)

115 How to use the European Convention for the Protection of Human Rights and Fundamental Freedoms in matters of reproductive law: the case law of the European Court of Human Rights. Guide
KRZYZANOWSKA-MIERZEWSKA, MAGDA. Warsaw, Federation for Women and Family Planning, ASTRA Network, 2004. 130 p.
The three-part guide contains an introduction to the system for protection of human rights under the European Convention on the Protection of Human Rights and Fundamental Freedoms. The second part covers proceedings before the court, including how to submit an application, general tips on procedure, essential elements of an application, legal representation, use of languages, hearings, settlements, judgements and Grand Chamber cases. The third part gives information on substantive rights relevant to reproductive and sexual health.
http://www.astra.org.pl/astra_guide.htm (accessed October 2005)

116 Health sector reform and reproductive health in Latin America and the Caribbean: strengthening the links
LANGER, A; NIGENDA, G.; CATINO, J. *Bulletin of the World Health Organization* 78(2000)5, p. 667-676 ISSN 0042-9686
Health sector reforms are taking place in different ways, at different speeds and with differing results in many Latin American countries and the Caribbean. Three regional workshops held in Mexico City, Quito and Brasilia in 1999 focused on issues of decentralization, changes in health services financing and the role of the private sector. These factors have not generally been well coordinated, resulting in overlapping policies and slow implementation. Conclusions and recommendations from the workshops propose a continuous dialogue at regional and country levels. The importance of participatory processes for monitoring progress is emphasized, as is the importance of the role of NGOs. The strengthening of local level capacity is important, to enable client input on the design and delivery of health services. Work with international aid organizations is required to develop practical methods of support for national health sector reform, with reproductive health as a priority. The implementation of health sector reform and reproductive health approaches should mutually reinforce each other, which requires changes at all levels of the health care system.
http://www.who.int/docstore/bulletin/pdf/2000/issue5/bu0560.pdf (accessed October 2005)
KIT Library shelf mark: K 1906-78(2000)5

annotated bibliography

117 Gendering prevention practices: a practical guide to working with gender in sexual safety and HIV/AIDS awareness education
LEWIS, JILL. Oslo, The Nordic Institute for Women's Studies and Gender Research (NIKK), 2003. 52 p. ISBN 82-7864-0157
Discussion of gender in any culture involves an exploration of popular beliefs, attitudes and expectations, looking at a society's traditions, culture, laws, etc. It also means increasing awareness of inherent inequalities in gendered sexual relations that endanger sexual safety and health. Group activities help to develop a critical literacy towards better sexual health education and HIV/AIDS prevention. The challenge is to encourage flexibility and open-minded reflection. The examples provided are workshop exercises used in many different countries, from Sierra Leone and the USA to Sweden, South Africa, England and Bosnia. They generated debate with men and women in different contexts and with widely differing roles, from teachers and students to members of the police and refugees, nurses and soldiers.
http://www.nikk.uio.no/forskning/nikk/living/publ/lft_ gendprevpract.pdf (accessed October 2005)

118 Gendering AIDS: women, men, empowerment, mobilization
LEWIS, MIRANDA. London, Voluntary Service Overseas (VSO), 2003. 53 p.
A decrease in the spread and impact of HIV/AIDS in South Africa, Namibia, India and Cambodia is not yet happening because of a failure to reduce inequalities between men and women. VSO-conducted research (2003) observes an overlap between lack of rights, gender inequalities and HIV/AIDS through experience among VSO partner organizations, people living with HIV/AIDS and women's and men's organizations. Key indicators include gender violence and the inability to discuss sex with partners, unequal property rights linked to stigmatism and limited work opportunities for women, predominantly female carers, unequal access to treatment and prevention information. A three-pronged approach recommends increasing men's involvement in activities to address HIV/AIDS and gender inequalities, empowering women by implementing women's rights, and addressing the immediate needs of women affected by HIV/AIDS as carers, sufferers of gender violence, and people required treatment for HIV/AIDS. Changes in policy and practice are needed at many levels of policy and practice. Recommendations include considering the needs of men who have sex with men, prioritizing training and support for staff in the public sector (police, doctors, nurses, social workers etc.), and providing access to accurate, easily understandable information for everyone.
http://www.vso.org.uk/Images/gendering_aids_tcm8-809.pdf (accessed October 2005)

119 Gender and health sector reform: analytical perspectives on African experience
MACKINTOSH, MAUREEN; TIBANDEBAGE, PAULA. Prepared for the UNRISD report Gender equality: striving for justice in an unequal world. Draft working document. May 7th, 2004. Geneva, United Nations Research Institute for Social Development (UNRISD), 2004. 42 p.
The state of women's health is not only defined by their sex and reproductive role, but by their general health and the effects of social, cultural and economic factors. More gender equity means eliminating discrimination against women and giving attention to women's differentiated health needs. An exploration of health sector reforms (HSRs), particularly in Africa, indicates that, in their current design, HSRs do not contribute to the objective of addressing, for example, the impact of HIV/AIDS on women and the elderly, and indeed may even be worsening the situation in some respects. Although reports such as the World Bank (1993) 'Investing in Health' document identify education, access to income and differentiated health needs as important issues for women, proposed reforms tend to overlook gender differences. The health sector itself is gendered, and as such reflects inequalities in staffing and priority-setting. An essential step towards achieving a lessening of the deprivation of poor women and relative disadvantages for women is therefore firstly an analysis of the gendered nature of institutions. Recommended proposals for reform design would ensure that the economic burden on women is not increased, that it would promote equality among health workers, involve both men and women in reform efforts, reduce the burden of work on (especially poor) women, ease access to health care and generally strengthen women's rights and status outside the health sector.
http://www.unrisd.org/80256B3C005BCCF9/httpNetIT FramePDF?ReadForm&parentunid=0461F951FA73D08 FC1256FE2003167CE&parentdoctype=paper&netitpath= 80256B3C005BCCF9/(httpAuxPages)/0461F951FA73D08 FC1256FE2003167CE/$file/mackinto.pdf (accessed October 2004)

120 Women's human rights related to health-care services in the context of HIV/AIDS
MACNAUGHTON, GILLIAN. *Health and Human Rights Working Paper Series 5*. London, International Centre for the Legal Protection of Human Rights (INTERIGHTS), 2004. 32 p.

gender and health: policy and practice

About 20 years ago, women and girls were in the minority of those infected by HIV/AIDS. They now account for 50% globally, even 58% in sub-Saharan Africa, the region most affected. In South Asia, twice as many women than men (aged 15-24) live with HIV/AIDS. Although in recent years the price of antiretrovirals (ARVs) has fallen radically in low-income countries, to US$132 per person per year, less than 300,000 of the 6 million who need this treatment are receiving it. An enormous increase in health-care services is necessary for delivery, with related HIV testing, counseling and perhaps life-long ARV treatment. The scale-up is bringing human rights issues to the fore which need to be addressed, especially for women and girls in developing countries. Different forms of gender inequality are intertwined. Women are often poorly informed about sexual matters in societies where children are socialized according to strongly gendered norms. Cultural norms and violence against women mean that they feel unable to negotiate safer sex with their partners. Economic and legal inequities prevent women's access to land, property, credit, employment and education, reinforcing economic dependence and vulnerability. Discrimination frequently occurs within the health-care system, including denial of treatment, HIV testing without consent and breaches of confidentiality with consequent social discrimination. It is possible to challenge human rights abuses, even where legislation is absent. An international commitment to human rights is essential to deal with HIV/AIDS globally, as recognized by the UN.
http://www.who.int/hhr/information/en/Series_5_womens healthcarerts_MacNaughtonFINAL.pdf (accessed October 2005)

121 Making safe motherhood a reality in West Africa: using indicators to programme for results
New York, NY, United Nations Population Fund (UNFPA), 2003. 36 p.
This report documents UNFPA's efforts to address maternal mortality using a strategic and practical evidence-based approach in a region where data has been scarce, and where too many women have died. Increasing access to emergency obstetric care is central to this approach.
http://www.unfpa.org/upload/lib_pub_file/149_filename_safemwestfrica.pdf (accessed October 2005)

122 Gendered communication among young people in Mexico: implications for sexual health interventions
MARSTON, C. *Social Science and Medicine* 59(2004)3, p. 445-456 ISSN 0277-9536

Effective communication between men and women can have a positive effect on sexual health. Gender affects communication in two ways. Firstly, social stereotypes can prohibit the expression of sexual desire on the part of women more than men. For example, women may feel they must say 'no' to sex even when they mean yes. Secondly, the manner in which men and women speak is also gendered, e.g., 'aggressive' men vs. 'passive' women. Language among young people in Mexico appears to reflect social context rather than actual behaviour. Health interventions that enhance communication between men and women should have a positive impact on sexual health. Research and interventions that do not address social pressures may reinforce communication barriers. The Gente Joven (Young People) programme in Mexico emphasizes respect for others, and creates contexts where men and women learn to interact and speak to each other about 'risky' topics in a safe environment.
KIT Library shelf mark: E 2085-59(2004)3

123 Maternal mortality update 2004 update 2004: ...delivering into good hands
New York, NY, United Nations Population Fund (UNFPA), 2004. 32 p.
In many developing countries, failing health systems and a lack of social and political commitment result in high maternal mortality. Nearly two-thirds of maternal deaths worldwide are due to five direct causes, all of which can be treated by a professional health worker. Maternal mortality ratio estimates are highest in Africa (830), followed by Asia (330), Oceania (240), Latin America and the Caribbean (190) and the developed countries (20). In sub-Saharan Africa, the risk of maternal death may be 1 in 16, compared to 1 in 2800 in developed countries. Adolescents are particularly at risk. Since so much of maternal mortality is avoidable, death during pregnancy or childbirth is a violation of women's rights to life and health, as well as a social injustice. Rights-based approaches promote the empowerment of women and support the possibility of safe delivery. Skilled attendance at birth is key to saving the lives of mothers and newborns. There is no single approach to improving skilled attendance, and strategies must be tailored to suit local contexts.
http://www.unfpa.org/upload/lib_pub_file/381_filename_mmupdate05_eng21.pdf (accessed October 2005)

annotated bibliography

124 Endangered youth? Youth, gender, and sexualities in urban Botswana
MCILWAINE, CATHY; DATTA, KAVITA. *Gender, Place and Culture* 11(2004)4, p. 483-512 ISSN 0966-369X
The article explores the construction of sexualities among young people in Botswana and how this is linked to awareness of the causes and effects of HIV/AIDS and teenage pregnancy. Identity is seen as a process of social constructionism. The construction of identity among the young is based largely on sex and sexualities due to the overwhelming importance of HIV/AIDS and teenage pregnancy in their lives. The discussion draws on empirical research from a pilot study in Gaborone using participatory urban appraisal methodologies. It elaborates on social constructionism in the context of interactions between youth, gender and sexualities. Familialization and individualization are critical aspects, producing conceptualizations of children and youth as dependents on the one hand, and of rights and entitlements on the other. The discussion highlights the need for recognition of the diversity of sexualities, being influenced by the dominant Tswana culture as well as other circumstances associated with public health campaigns. Sexualities need to be seen as a holistic contruct rather than a public health issue, because of the impact of social, cultural and economic circumstances. There is a need for renewed debate on youth agency and empowerment. Only by engaging with young people as active agents of change will further progress be made in addressing HIV / AIDS and teenage pregnancy crises in Botswana.
KIT Library shelf mark: H 2448-11(2004)4

125 Mental health
Gender and Health Research Series. Geneva, Department of Gender, Women and Health (GWH), World Health Organization (WHO), 2004. 40 p. refs. ISBN 92-4-159253-2
Although there is little difference between men and women in terms of the prevalence of mental health disorders, some disorders are clearly more common among women and others among men. Gender-based factors such as unemployment, marital arrangements and suicide methods have a significant relationship to depression, substance abuse and (attempted) suicide rates. There are also significant gender differences in the impact and outcome of disorders that have no significant gender prevalence. Gender appears to be a factor in health-seeking behaviour, treatment and care, the stigma attached to mental disorders, and position within the family. There are numerous overlaps between reproductive and mental health, for example in the areas of postnatal depression, rape, still births and miscarriage, infertility, etc. There is as yet little systematic research into links between men's reproductive and sexual health and mental although, although there is evidence to suggest them. Recommendations for future research suggest the inclusion of both men and women, results broken down by sex, measurement of gender factors in the cause, course, treatment-seeking patterns, impact and outcome of mental disorders, the impact of socioeconomic variables from a gendered perspective, and the inclusion of gendered mental health factors in other gender and health research. The integration of mental health concerns into gender and health research would be of mutual benefit to researchers.
http://www.who.int/gender/documents/en/mentalhealthlo w.pdf (accessed October 2005)

126 What about boys? A literature review on the health and development of adolescent boys
MIKULENCAK, MANDY (ed.). *WHO/FCH/CAH/00.7*. Geneva, Department of Child and Adolescent Health and Development, World Health Organization (WHO), 2000. 58 p. refs.
Generalizations about adolescent boys do not take into account that they are a heterogeneous population. Some of them face risks and have needs that have not previously been considered, or are socialized in ways that lead to violence and discrimination against women. Some comparison between males and females may be inevitable, but should not polarize the debate. The challenge is to examine the specific needs of boys in ways that promote greater gender equity, and look at the positive contribution of boys to their families and societies. Research shows that adolescent boys, like girls, have gender-specific potentials and risks.
http://www.promundo.org.br/materia/resources/files/ download/WhatAboutBoys.pdf (accessed October 2005)

127 Gender equity and socioeconomic inequality: a framework for the patterning of women's health
MOSS, NANCY E. *Social Science and Medicine* 54(2002)5, p. 649-661 ISSN 0277-9536
Health issues tend to be examined within two different paradigms, gender and socioeconomics. The proposed multi-level framework brings them together for the purpose of improving understanding of physical and mental health effects on women. Socioeconomic and gender inequality affect women's health in multiple

ways, and the proposed model explores various geopolitical and cultural factors at country levels, as well as women's roles in reproduction and production at household and individual levels. These factors include geography and history, policies and services, legal rights and organizations, as well as cultural influences and socio-demographic characteristics at home and at work. The paper proposes a variety of approaches for extended research and policy making for the promotion of gender and socioeconomic equity and women's health. The proposed combined framework in this paper can be applied to health services irrespective of geography. The intention is to understand the similarities and differences in women's health issues so as to be able to develop effective policies for their greater well being.
KIT Library shelf mark: E 2085-54(2002)5

128 Act now: a resource guide for young women on HIV/AIDS
MSIMANG, SISONKE; WILSON, SHAMILLAH. New York, NY, United Nations Development Fund for Women (UNIFEM), 2002. 47 p. ISBN 0-912917-64-4
An online discussion forum for young women generates large numbers of messages from a total of 500 participants in a three-week period. The documented forum reviews discussions of HIV/AIDS in relation to youth and gender, emerging challenges and successes, especially for young women, and ways in which young people can participate in approaches to gender and youth issues in HIV/AIDS programmes. Recommendations for AIDS programmes, best practices, and guidelines are provided for the planning and execution of HIV/AIDS workshops for young women.
http://www.awid.org/publications/ActNow.pdf (accessed October 2005)

129 Gender-based barriers to primary health care provision in Pakistan: the experience of female providers
MUMTAZ, ZUBIA. *Health Policy and Planning* 18(2003)3, p. 261-269, refs. ISSN 0268-1080
Female health and family planning workers in Pakistan face the same gender constraints that necessitate their work at community level. Recruitment, training and retention of these women is made difficult by abusive management structures, disrespect from male colleagues, lack of sensitivity to gender-based cultural constraints on women, conflict between domestic and work responsibilities and poor infrastructural support. Links between women's public and private lives and between class and gender hierarchies have

an impact on how women experience the employment situation. Restricted mobility and constraints on male-female interaction are further factors that inhibit improvements in heath services. Female health workers in some communities experience low social status, poor working conditions and sexual exploitation. Female employees need to challenge the existing system, with the support of men in senior management positions who are sympathetic to gender-sensitive organizational development. Formal gender training is also necessary to create collective self-awareness and the desirability of change.
KIT Library shelf mark: E 2772-18(2003)3

130 'I never go anywhere': extricating the links between women's mobility and uptake of reproductive health services in Pakistan
MUMTAZ, ZUBIA; SALAWY, SARAH. *Social Science and Medicine* 60(2005)8, p. 1751-1765, refs. ISSN 0277-9536
Women's mobility is an important factor in their access to health care and improvement of health. Independent mobility may also improve health indirectly because of the potential for greater exposure to information, the development of interpersonal skills and greater self-confidence. However, this view is influenced by Western feminism. The question of women's mobility in Pakistan is complex, depending on interacting factors of class and gender hierarchies. Poor women travelling alone are associated with lower prestige and susceptibility to sexual violence. In the current situation, it is not prudent for Pakistani women to travel unaccompanied, particularly if pregnant, when seeking reproductive health services. The need for reproductive health care and increasing women's social resources are more important issues.
KIT Library shelf mark: E 2085-60(2005)8

131 Health sector reforms and sexual reproductive health services: lessons and gaps emerging from the Initiative for Sexual and Reproductive Rights in Health Reforms
MURTHY, RANJANI K.; DE PINHO, HELEN; RAVINDRAN, SUNDARI T.K.; ROMERO, MARIANA. Paper prepared for the Technical consultation of WHO on Health sector reform: developing the evidence base, Geneva, 30 November-2 December 2004. Women's Health Project, 2005. 28 p.
The Rights and Reforms Initiative began in 2002 to bridge the gap in understanding between neo-liberal reformers including the World Bank, USAID and others and sexual and reproductive health rights (SRHR) advocates. It is led by

SRHR advocates from Asia, Africa and Latin America, who have reviewed six crucial elements of health sector reforms: financing, public-private interactions, priority-setting, decentralization, integration of services and accountability. The findings of the Initiative are that reforms have not solved the problems it intended to solve, and that to some extent, availability, affordability, equity and quality have been reduced. Gaps in knowledge need to be addressed for reforms to be effective. Specific themes for research are proposed, including the inter-relationship of different elements of reforms, the impact of different social, political and economic contexts, the impact of reforms on SRH services over time, and monitoring mechanisms. An assessment of positive outcomes in some countries is required, so as to ascertain what global and local solutions may be required outside the health sector, in order to address problems in health systems in developing countries.

http://www.wits.ac.za/whp/rightsandreforms/docs/global overviewdraft.pdf (accessed October 2005)

132 A decade after Cairo: women's health in a free market economy

NAIR, S; KIRBAT, P.; SEXTON, S. *Briefing 31*. Dorset, The Corner House, 2004. 36 p.
The current decline in maternal health and reproductive health and rights contradicts the resolutions made at the International Conference on Population and Development (ICPD). Ten years on, there are still 600,000 maternal deaths every year, 95% of them in sub-Saharan Africa and Asia, and 18 million women suffer preventable complications from pregnancy or childbirth. The struggle for reproductive health and rights means the abolition of gender, class, racial and ethnic injustice. Macroeconomic and religious fundamentalist activities that perpetuate gender, race and class inequalities stop others from achieving reproductive and sexual rights. Women cannot exercise their reproductive rights if other rights are not respected; more attention must be paid to specific geographic and cultural contexts. Success in improving reproductive rights is greatest where there are popular movements as well as NGO and governmental programmes, such as those in Brazil, the Philippines, India, South Africa and Peru. Networking and appropriate alliances could help such movements. Feminist activists are paving the way for the incorporation of reproductive and sexual rights within larger social contexts.

http://www.thecornerhouse.org.uk/pdf/briefing/31cairo.pdf (accessed October 2005)

133 Accelerating progress towards achieving the MDG to improve maternal health: a collection of promising approaches

NANDA, GEETA; SWITLICK, KIMBERLY; LULE ELIZABETH. *Health, Nutrition and Population (HNP) Discussion Paper*. Washington, DC, World Bank, 2005. 174 p.
Global promising approaches can be useful in the improvement of maternal health programming. Effective programmes must be implemented that are relevant to specific countries' setting, policies and resources in order to scale up efforts to achieve the Millennium Development Goal (MDG) to improve maternal health. Evidence-based knowledge and strategies are available. While not all of them have yet been rigorously evaluated, they are documented and disseminated to share knowledge and illustrate recent and innovative efforts in the field. An introduction to the approaches looks at the magnitude of the problem, the rationale for investing in maternal health, and key technical interventions. The latter include emergency obstetric care, management of unsafe abortion and family planning services. Different approaches consider such factors as government policies and actions, health systems and financing, access to health services, building capacity, the quality of care, and community involvement. Monitoring and advancing progress is discussed as well as work with partnerships and collaborations.

http://www-wds.worldbank.org/servlet/WDSContent Server/WDSP/IB/2005/04/13/000090341_20050413093654/ Rendered/PDF/319690HNP0Nandl1ingProgress01public1 .pdf (accessed October 2005)

134 Women's nutrition throughout the life cycle and in the context of HIV and AIDS: training of trainers module

NTOMBELA, N.; STONE-JIMENEZ, M.; ROSS, J.; MARTIN, L. Washington, DC, Academy for Educational Development, Linkages Project, 2005. 108 p.
Training health workers on nutrition throughout the complete life-cycle of women includes providing guidance on nutritional status, causes of malnutrition, effects of malnutrition, consequences of inadequate weight and height, and micro-nutrient deficiencies. The relationships between nutrition and HIV infection are covered, with specific sections on field practice. training is based on behaviour change communication (BCC) using a range of methods including demonstration, practice,

gender and health: policy and practice

discussion, case studies and role play. The emphasis is on participation.
http://www.linkagesproject.org/media/publications/Training%20Modules//Womens-Nutrition_module_May_05.pdf (accessed October 2005)

135 Making schools a safe horizon for girls: a training manual on preventing sexual violence against girls in schools
ODHIAMBO, M.A.; MAGANYA, J. ActionAid International Kenya and the Cradle – the Children's Foundation (Child's Rights Advisory, Documentation and Legal Center), 2004. 146 p.
The safety of girls is a serious issue in schools, where teachers are increasing reported to perpetrate sexual harassment against girl pupils. There have been cases of pregnancy and early marriage. Yet children are afraid to report harassment or violation by teachers, who are a symbol of authority. Consequently, they suffer in silence or drop out of school. Training for teachers, education officials, inspectors and parents in the prevention and handling of sexual abuse covers problem analysis; understanding children and gender dynamics; the rights of children and the impact of childhood experiences on later life; guidance on identifying abused children in schools and how to help and protect them, and the legal situation; counseling and action planning. The training manual provides guidelines for the preparation and execution of training by means of workshops.
http://www.iicrd.org/cap/files/SafeHorizonsforGirls_0.pdf (accessed October 2005)

136 The prevention of unsafe abortion in Africa
OKONOFUA, FRDAY E.; HESSINI, LEILA; WOLF, MERRILL. *African Journal of Reproductive Health* 8(2004)1, special issue ISSN 1118-4841
Most of Africa's 54 countries have restrictive abortion laws, resulting in nearly five million unsafe abortions annually. While abortion law reform is steadily progressing since the 1960s, liberalised laws do not necessarily mean expanded access for women. This is due to various factors including shortages of trained providers and equipment, and US reversals of commitments on funding for sexual and reproductive rights health services. A critical first step in addressing the problem is to break the silence surrounding the issue in scientific as well as political and domestic contexts. The handling of unsafe abortion requires preventive measures at primary, secondary and tertiary levels. Primary measures concern the prevention of unwanted pregnancies leading to abortion. Secondary measures relate to safe termination of unwanted pregnancies, and tertiary measures concern post-abortion care. Health systems must be trained and equipped to make safe abortion services available. Women need to be able to make independent and safe reproductive choices for the sake of their and their families' future. Shifting power relations to rebalance gender inequities, providing access to technological medical equipment, and appropriate sexuality education for young people are all requisites for the reduction of unsafe abortion and high levels of maternal morbidity and mortality. A case study of the introduction of medical abortion in Tunisia provides an example of a successful intervention approach.
KIT Library shelf mark: H 2491-8(2004)1

137 Gender and equity in health sector reform: a review of the literature
ONYANGO, CHRISTINE. Washington, DC, Pan American Health Organization (PAHO), 2001. 42 p. refs.
Increasing concern about the interaction of health sector reform and gender is partly a result of UN conferences in the 1990s putting women's human rights at the centre of health policies. Evidence from around the world demonstrates inequality in the health status of women and men. This review looks at the assumptions behind links between gender and the use of health services, the gender impact of activities, reforms, decentralization and privatization. There is also a review of the gender impact of measures to improve the functioning of national Ministries of Health. New financing mechanisms are explored in terms of the introduction of user fees, community financing schemes, and social and private insurance schemes. Managed care, as implemented in the USA and subsequently, Latin America, is discussed. In conclusion, gender impacts of health sector reforms are seen to predominantly concern decentralization and the privatization of financing and services. Empirical data is needed to help remedy the negative gender impact of health sector reform in progress, and prevent it where reforms are beginning.
http://www.paho.org/English/DPM/GPP/GH/ReformLitReview.pdf (accessed October 2005)

137a What evidence is there about the effects of health care reforms on gender equity, particularly in health?
ÖSTLIN, PIROSKA. Geneva, World Health organization (WHO), 2005. 15 p.
In most countries the pressure for health care reform is aimed at improving the efficiency, equity and effectiveness of the health sector.

Emerging evidence shows that health care reforms can affect men and women differently, as a consequence of their different positions as users and producers of health care. This review assesses the impact of four key health reforms, decentralization, financing, privatisation and priority setting, on gender equity in health. The literature reveals that the consequences of health care reforms for gender equity, particularly in health care, are seldom taken into consideration when designing fundamental changes to health care systems. Policy considerations are suggested.
http://www.euro.who.int/Document/E87674.pdf
(accessed November 2005)

138 Paying attention to gender and poverty in health research: content and process issues
ÖSTLIN, PIROSKA; SEN, GITA; GEORGE, ASHA. *Bulletin of the World Health Organization* 82(2004)10, p. 740-745 ISSN 0042-9686
Poverty and gender are the most consistently important indicators of health inequity. Poverty is known to cause ill health, but ill health can itself cause poverty. In rural India, over 80% of cases of poverty were found to result to a critical extent from poor health and health-related expenses. Improvements in average health status in the second half of the 20th century have led to a dramatic decline in mortality, but the improvements are not equally distributed. There are significant gaps in the content and processes of health research with regard to gender and poverty. Research needs to recognize the possible gender differences in the risk factors, causes. consequences and management of diseases, and in health outcomes. It is important to understand the interaction of such factors as poverty, race, caste, sexual orientation and gender. Two of the most important triggers of decisive national policy relate to health research: scientific evidence, and alliances and communication between policy makers, scientists, health professionals, NGOs and the public.
http://www.who.int/bulletin/volumes/82/10/en/740.pdf
(accessed October 2005)

139 Gender and mental health research in developing countries
PATEL, VIKRAM. Paper presented at the Global Forum for Health Research, Arusha, November 2002. 9 p.
It is thought that less than 10% of all health research in developing countries studies non-communicable diseases, and that of these, less than 10% focus on mental health. By examining the relationships between gender and mental health, and reproductive health and mental health, it could be possible to generate data that are relevant to broader public health issues and programmes. Depression and anxiety disorders are the most common psychological illnesses in the world. These disorders are often associated with poverty and lower income groups. Although many sufferers from depression are undiagnosed and untreated, surveys indicate that the numbers of women out-number men by almost 2 to 1. This varies from place to place: in Nigeria, men are in the majority, but in Santiago de Chile the female-male ratio is 4.7:1. Women with mental illness also tend to experience greater discrimination than men. Since women's health goes beyond reproductive issues, mental health issues and needs should be integrated with other priorities.
http://www.globalforumhealth.org/forum_6/sessions/2wednesday/3GMentalHealthPatelGenderFull.rtf
(accessed October 2005)

140 Population, reproductive rights and reproductive health with special reference to HIV/AIDS: a concise report
ST/ESA/SER.A 214. New York, NY, Department of Economic and Social Affairs, United Nations, 2004. 81 p. 92-1-151373-1
Reproductive health and rights cover issues related to entry into reproductive life, reproductive behaviour, family planning, abortion, maternal mortality and morbidity, sexually transmitted infections, HIV/AIDS, and reproductive rights. Different phases and conditions of life have implications for reproductive health. Child survival is linked to mothers' health, for example. Major risks attend premature entry into sexual relationships, multiple partners, early childbearing, and unsafe abortion. HIV/AIDS and sexually transmitted infections pose a major threat. In women, menopause can trigger alterations in the skeletal and cardiovascular systems. In men, prostate glad tumours are relatively common. Much progress has been made since the ICPD in Cairo in 1994 and the subsequent Beijing Conference on Women to establish the basis for reproductive rights, but much remains to be done. It is likely that reproductive rights will continue to play an important role in population policies in years to come.

141 Preventing violence: a guide to implementing the recommendations of the World report on violence and health
Geneva, World Health Organization (WHO), 2004. 92 p. ISBN 92-4-159207-9

The core components of interpersonal violence prevention activities involve multiple sectors in an action plan at national level. Conceptual aspects concern the general principles in implementation; policy issues cover relationships to policy instruments and development processes within the health and other sectors, the use of existing and the creation of new policies for better prevention, and for victim services and support. Action Steps provide practical suggestions for implementation, with checklists and templates for evaluation. Both multi-sector involvement and clear leadership are important for the success of efforts at all levels to prevent violence.

http://whqlibdoc.who.int/publications/2004/9241592079. pdf (accessed October 2005)

142 Addressing the reproductive health needs and rights of young people since ICPD: the contribution of UNFPA and IPPF. Synthesis report
PRICE, NEIL. Bonn, Federal Ministry for Economic Cooperation and Development (BMZ), 204. 80 p. Includes CD-ROM
The synthesis report evaluates good practice and strategic lessons arising from the contribution of the United Nations Population Fund (UNFPA) and the International Planned Parenthood Federation (IPPF) to the reproductive rights and health needs of young people. Following details of the background, methodological approach and report structure, the synthesis report summaries the progress achieved since the International Conference on Population and Development (ICPD) in 1994. Summary data are provided for the countries evaluated: Bangladesh, Burkina Faso, Egypt, Nicaragua, Tanzania and Vietnam. The evaluation provides country-specific information on programmes, contexts and strategies, institutional capacity and arrangements, policy developments and reforms, and reproductive health services and information. Conclusions from the evaluations are followed by recommendations for UNFPA, IPPF and affiliates, and for collaborative action between UNFPA and Family Planning Associations at country level.
KIT Library shelf mark: G 04-183

143 Programme planning materials and training resources: a compendium
New York, United Nations Population Fund (UNFPA), Margaret Sanger Center International, 2004. 308 p. ISBN 0-89714-728-6
With over a billion young people worldwide on the verge of adulthood, it is important to focus more on working with youth on sexual and reproductive health issues, especially with regard to the prevention of HIV. The essential elements for successful youth-focused programmes cover guiding principles on rights and equity-based concepts; programme strategies that address service, policy and education needs; and administrative and managerial capacities for the development of efficient, sustainable programmes. The Compendium brings together materials focusing specifically on HIV prevention for young people, identified through a mapping process that sources programme planning documents worldwide. Most of the materials were designed for use in a variety of cultural settings. Regionally-specific documents predominantly refer to projects in Africa, followed by Asia and the Pacific, Latin America and the Caribbean and North America in nearly equal numbers. The majority of the documents are in English, although there are some in Spanish, French and Nepali, and date from 2000 to 2003. The materials are mostly training manuals, modules and curricula for the implementation of training and workshops in HIV prevention programmes. There are also reports on case studies and interventions, and guidelines.

http://www.unfpa.org/upload/lib_pub_file/367_filename_ compendium.pdf (accessed October 2005)

144 Promise of equality: gender equity, reproductive health and the Millennium Development Goals
New York, NY, United Nations Population Fund (UNFPA), 2005. 128 p. ISBN 0-89714-750-2
This report explores the degree to which the global community has fulfilled pledges made to the world's most impoverished and marginalized peoples. It tracks progress, exposes shortfalls and examines the links between poverty, gender equality, human rights, reproductive health, conflict and violence against women and girls. It also examines the relationship between gender discrimination and the scourge of HIV/AIDS. It identifies the vulnerabilities and strengths of history's largest cohort of young people and highlights the critical role they play in development. The MDGs constitute a promise by the world's leaders to find solutions to challenges that plague humanity. The eight goals range from halving extreme poverty to tackling the problem of maternal mortality, and reversing the HIV/AIDS epidemically by 2015. As well as pinpointing an actual date for their achievement, the MDGs include one goal, promote gender equality and empower women, that is critical to the success of the other seven. Although the goal of universal access to reproductive health by 2015, agreed at the 1994 International Conference

on Population and Development (ICPD), was not explicitly included in the MDGs, investments in this area are now considered essential to their achievement

http://www.unfpa.org/swp/2005/pdf/en_swp05.pdf (accessed October 2005)
KIT Library shelf mark: K 2562-(2005)

145 Female genital mutilation: a guide to laws and policies worldwide

RAHMAN, ANIKA; TOUBIA, NAHID. London, Zed Books in association with CRLP and RAINBO, 2000. 249 p. ISBN 1-85649-773-9
A report is given on female circumcision (FC) as practised in 28 African countries and a sampling of 13 countries with immigrant populations from countries where FC is practised. Part I contains an overview of the background and history of FC and related health and medical issues. It places the subject within an international legal framework, containing recommendations for legal and policy measures to be taken by governments. The report suggests a solution to the problem of FC through the implementation of human rights treaties. Part II contains 41 national profiles indicating the pertinent international treaties, national laws and other measures in force in each country. The report is the result of research carried out by the CRLP and RAINBO using Demographic and Health Surveys in 7 African countries, UN reports and information provided by NGOs and government ministries in the profiled countries.
KIT Library shelf mark: P 00-1236

146 Reaching men to improve reproductive health for all: implementation guide

Prepared by Johns Hopkins Bloomberg School of Public Health/Center for Communication Programs. Washington, DC, Interagency Gender Working Group (IGWG), US Agency for International Development (USAID), 2003. 142 p.
This implementation guide presents examples of how to develop, implement, and evaluate reproductive health (RH) programmes that involve men with a gender-sensitive perspective, i.e. in ways that promote gender equity and improve health outcomes for men and women. These programme examples were presented at the conference, Reaching men to improve reproductive health for all, held in Dulles, Virginia in September 2003. A gender-sensitive perspective on reproductive health programmes involves working with men to promote gender equity and improve health outcomes for men and women. The importance of male involvement, as sexual partners, fathers and decision makers, is established. Programmes with (especially young)

men indicate that they are willing to change their attitudes, beliefs and behaviour. They are open to ways of expressing their masculinity that do not rely on virility and violence. Men can help reduce maternal mortality and women's higher vulnerability to HIV. Programmes provide men with information and education on sexual and reproductive health issues, reducing the risk of STIs and HIV infection, and correcting misconceptions. Men can be reached in various contexts: at their place of employment, through entertainment, or in the community; through trade unions, the armed forces, schools and the media. Community members, traditional and local leaders can be trained as promoters to inform others about reproductive health. The implementation guide is also available on the Web and on CD-ROM.
http://www.jhuccp.org/igwg/guide/guide.pdf (accessed October 2005)

147 Improving reproductive health care within the context of district health services: a hands-on manual for planners and managers

REERINK, IETJE H.; CAMPBELL, BRUCE BENNER. Amsterdam, KIT (Royal Tropical Institute), 2004. 155 p. ISBN 9068321544
This hands-on manual is designed to help district health staff in systematically planning, implementing, monitoring and reviewing sexual and reproductive health (SRH) activities, as part of the overall district health plan. It is designed for individuals, alone or as part of a team, who have responsibility for the planning and management of SRH and primary health care services in the district. The manual guides the user through different stages of the management cycle, from review of existing services to strategic planning for additional or new activities, implementation, monitoring, performance review and evaluation.
http://smartsite.kit.nl/net/KIT_Publicaties_output/ showfile.aspx?a=tblFiles&b=FileID&c=FileName&d= TheFile&e=457 (accessed October 2005)
KIT Library shelf mark: G 04-9; G 04-18; Br N 03-293 (CD-ROM); Br N 03-304 (CD-ROM)

148 Re-thinking differences and rights in sexual and reproductive health: a training manual for health care providers

Durham, NC, Family Health International (FHI), 2005
The training package presented here is designed to promote an approach to sexual and reproductive health care that recognizes different needs and perspectives within a context of respect for the rights and dignity of men and women. It includes a conceptual framework and a

guide for training activities. The package was completed in 1998 and was immediately put to use and tested in training sessions in La Paz and Santa Cruz, Bolivia. It was well received and the participatory application process generated modifications, primarily in the exercises and examples given in the four modules. The package in its original form serves as a prototype and will be a useful resource to support training efforts in other cultural settings. For this reason the document has been translated from Spanish to English and is made widely available.

http://www.fhi.org/en/RH/Training/trainmat/rethinkDiff/index.htm (accessed October 2005)

149 Report of the Consultative Meeting to finalize a gender-sensitive core set of leading health indicators, 1-3 August 2004, Kobe, Japan
WHO/WKC/SYM/05.1. Kobe, World Health Organization (WHO) Centre for Health Development (WHO Kobe Centre), 2005. 11 p.
The objectives of the consultation and the rationale for using a comprehensive gender-sensitive core set of leading health indicators are outlined. The Consultative Meeting reaffirmed the desire to build on data for indicators already included in major reporting systems (such as reporting systems established in the context of WHO, MDGs and United Nations Common Country Assessment) and minimize the imposition of new requirements for collecting new data. However, it was also recognized that there are deficiencies in reporting systems for current indicators, and that some data collection systems would need to be adjusted if key dimensions of gender equity and health were to be addressed. The agreed set of indicators agreed upon during the meeting comprises 36 indicators in total, with 11 on health status, 13 on determinants of health and 11 on health systems performance. This set is considered as a potentially effective tool for policy advisers, decision makers and strategic planners. Advocates could also use this tool, provided that they are fully aware of the meaning and significance of the data. They should therefore be involved in the processes of reporting, analysis and reflection.
http://www.who.or.jp/library/cm_report.pdf (accessed October 2005)

150 Resource pack on gender and HIV/AIDS
Geneva and Amsterdam, UNAIDS Inter-Agency Task team on Gender & HIV/AIDS and KIT (Royal Tropical Institute), 2005. 110 p. ISBN 9241590394
The resource pack sets out the status of the AIDS epidemic globally and how it links with gender-based inequality and inequity. It analyses the impact of gender relations on the different aspects of the HIV/AIDS epidemic and makes recommendations for effective programme and policy options. It includes a review paper for expert consultation entitled 'Integrating gender into HIV/AIDS Programmes' prepared by Geeta Rao Gupta, Daniel Whelan and Keera Allendorf, International Center for Research on Women (ICRW) on behalf of the WHO, and 16 fact sheets with concise information on gender related aspects of HIV/AIDS, prepared by different UN agencies involved. The Operational Guide, developed by KIT (Royal Tropical Institute), seeks to give guidance to development practitioners by providing a coherent conceptual framework from a gender and rights perspective and a set of guidelines, checklists and tools for programme implementation.
http://smartsite.kit.nl/net/KIT_Publicaties_output/publication_details.aspx?ItemID=1868 (accessed October 2005)

151 A rights-based approach to reproductive health
DAHLQUIST,. KRISTIN; KIRSHBAUM, JACK; KOLS, ADRIENNE. In: *Outlook* 20(2003)4, 8 p.
ISSN 0737-3732
A rights-based approach can provide tools to analyze the causes of health problems and inequities in health service delivery and influence health programmes and policies by placing reproductive health in a broader context. Many of the human rights defined in international human rights' treaties since 1965 have implications for reproductive health care. A rights-based approach to reproductive health is powerful because all human rights are universal, inalienable, indivisible and interdependent. These qualities mean that local cultural or religious traditions cannot be used as an excuse not to respect and protect all of women's rights, including their reproductive rights. Women's reproductive rights cannot be realized independently of their broader human rights, e.g. the right to freedom from poverty and the right to work. The benefits of a rights-based approach include the ethical framework provided for health practitioners, increased pressure on authorities to improve public health, raised visibility and thus urgency, empowerment through rights education, improved effectiveness of health interventions, wider awareness of gender issues and other societal factors that influence reproductive health. Effective action on reproduction health requires an integrated approach that draws on the related fields of ethics, law and human rights. Collaborative

annotated bibliography

153

programmes can address the social, cultural, economic, legal and policy factors affecting people's reproductive health, as well as other health concerns.
http://www.path.org/files/EOL_20_4_dec03.pdf (accessed October 2005)

152 Working with young men to promote sexual and reproductive health
RIVERS, KIM; AGGLETON, PETER. Highfield, Safe Passages to Adulthood Programme, University of Southampton, 2002. 37 p.
Young men present a number of opportunities for work to promote sexual and reproductive health. The Safe Passages to Adulthood programme organized a meeting to discuss such opportunities with researchers and practitioners across the world. Discussion took place over three days. As a result of the meeting, this summary and guide has been produced. It includes a number of illustrative case studies of the work of the projects, a discussion of key issues raised, and guidelines for work with young men.
http://www.socstats.soton.ac.uk/cshr/pdf/guidelines/ workingwithmen.pdf (accessed October 2005)

153 Generation dialogue about FGM and HIV/AIDS: method, experiences in the field and impact assessment
VAN ROENNE, ANNA. Eschborn, Deutsche Gesellschaft für Technische Zusammenarbeit (GTZ) and Federal Ministry for Economic Cooperation and Development (BMZ), 2005. 24 p.
The generation dialogue approach, field-tested in Guinea in 2003, was introduced following recognition of the ineffectiveness of previous approaches to the abandonment to female genital cutting (FGC). In 1999, Guinea had the highest rate of FGC in the world (98%). Since many were aware of the harmful effects of the practice, open debate was needed to discover the hidden factors for its continuance. The dialogue method, an integral part of a range of activities to encourage reflection, listening and dialogue in the community, is based on personal narrative in a respectful and enabling environment. Proposed changes are aligned with the people's own concepts, imagery and metaphors. The topics for dialogue are not dictated, but arise out of meetings between two generations. Older people contribute confidently on the subjects of traditional values and stories from the past, and current priority issues such as HIV/AIDS surface naturally. The dialogue schedule consists of two consecutive workshops linked by a one-month practical phase. The methods use the African oral tradition. In Guinea, for example, social and moral education takes place through the use of

proverbs, folk songs and dances. Exercises using brainstorming and group Q&A sessions function to encourage dialogues that the participants might otherwise never have, e.g. about differences in power between the generations. Generational differences in communication patterns may have been influenced by the dialogue approach. The results of a control survey showed significantly more communication between parents and children about sexual morality, HIV/AIDS and about genital mutilation, and improved family relationships.
http://www.afronets.kabissa.org/docs/GD-summary-report.pdf (accessed October 2005)

154 Safe abortion: technical and policy guidance for health systems
Geneva, World Health Organization (WHO), 2003. 110 p. ISBN 92-4-159034-3
Unsafe abortion is recognized as a major public health concern. It is a major contributor to maternal mortality and morbidity. Yet safe abortion services are frequently unavailable, even when it is legal to provide them. An enabling policy environment would ensure that eligible women have access to good-quality abortion services. Policies and programmes should make timely service provision accessible, ensure public knowledge of the law, and eliminate hindrances, unnecessary procedures and excessive restrictions. A 1999 Special Session of the UN reviewed progress made towards implementation of the 1994 Programme of Action of the International Conference on Population and Development in Cairo. The governments of the world then pledged their commitment to reduce the need for abortion through expanded and improved family planning services. The WHO technical and policy guidance publication provides an in-depth overview of safe abortion services and clinical care, guidelines for putting services in place, legal and policy considerations, and recommendations for removing barriers. It is intended for use by health professionals and others working to reduce maternal mortality and morbidity.
http://www.who.int/reproductive-health/publications/ safe_abortion/safe_abortion.pdf (accessed October 2005)

155 Reconciling cost recovery with health equity concerns in a context of gender inequality and poverty: findings from a new family health initiative in Bangladesh
SCHULER, SIDNEY RUTH; BATES, LISA; ISLAM, KHAIRUL. International Family Planning Perspectives 28(2002)4, p. 196-204 ISSN 0190-3187

gender and health: policy and practice

Changes in the delivery of family planning and other basic health services in Bangladesh emphasize quality, but entail higher costs for clients. The tension between a mandate to provide services to the poor while recovering costs presents difficulties for clinic staff. Results from surveys carried out in 1997 underlying the report reveal confusion among clients due to insufficient information as to government-subsidized and donated medication, lack of clarity about fee waivers and credit availability, and the complexities facing NGOs. The lack of transparency regarding credit and fee exemptions may even have forced poor women and children to forego health care. In Bangladesh, cultural norms such as reliance on personal connections, restrictions on women's mobility and lack of access to family money have meant that the impact of new health service delivery policies have not functioned as expected.
KIT Library shelf mark: H 1795-28(2002)4

156 Engendering international health: the challenge of equity
SEN, GITA; GEORGE, ASHA; ÖSTLIN, PIROSKA (eds). Cambridge, MA, MIT, 2002. 453 p. refs. ISBN 0-262-69273-2
This publication presents the work of leading researchers on gender equity in international health. Growing economic inequalities reinforce social injustice, stall health gains, and deny good health to many. In particular, gender biases in health research and policy institutions combine with a lack of well-articulated and accessible evidence to downgrade the importance of gender perspectives in health. The book's central premise is that unless public health changes direction, it cannot effectively address the needs of those who are most marginalized, many of whom are women. Evidence and analysis are offered for both low- and high-income countries, providing a gender and health analysis cross-cut by a concern for other markers of social equity, such as class and race. Approaches and agendas that incorporate, but go beyond, commonly acknowledge issues relating to women's health are detailed, and gender and equity analysis is brought into the heart of the debates that dominate international health policy.
KIT Library shelf mark: P 02-1575

157 Sex work and HIV/AIDS: technical update
UNAIDS Best Practice Collection. Technical Update. Geneva, Joint United Nations Programme on HIV/AIDS (UNAIDS), 2002. 20 p. ISBN 92-9173-159-5

This Technical Update focuses on the challenge in the protection of those involved in sex work and discusses the key elements of various interventions. Successful HIV/AIDS prevention and care programmes for those involved in sex work use a mix of strategies. Effective strategies that have been identified to date include promotion of safer sexual behaviour among sex workers, clients and institutions or groups associated with sex workers, such as police and sex workers' partners; promotion and availability of STI prevention and care services and outreach work that includes health, social and legal services. Current HIV/AIDS prevention programmes involving sex work are sometimes limited in coverage, inclusion and coordination of stakeholders, and long-term effectiveness and sustainability. Considerations to be taken into account when developing, implementing, monitoring and evaluating programmes are suggested, including the active involvement of sex workers themselves in all phases of project development, implementation and evaluation.
http://www.unaids.org/html/pub/Publications/IRC-pub02/JC705-SexWork-TU_en_pdf.pdf (accessed October 2005)

158 Sex work and HIV in Asia: MAP report 2005
ACHARYA, LAXMI BILAS; BARDON, JEANINE; BROWN, TIM; HARMON, KELLY SAFREED; HERSEY, SARA; JITTHAI, NIGOON; MALLICK, PARVEZ SAZZAD; MORINEAU, GUY; PISANI, ELIZABETH; WINITDHAMA, GANRAWI. Monitoring the AIDS Pandemic (MAP), 2005. 32 p.
People who buy or sell sex may be exposed to HIV and other sexual infections. Even when knowledge about and access to condoms is provided, some sex workers and many of their clients refuse to use them. Some Asian countries have recently seen rises in HIV infection rates among sex workers, which appear to stem from the spread of HIV among injecting drug users. The right prevention services can change the course of HIV epidemics in Asia. Successful prevention is seen to address the specific behaviour that cause most infections, provide large-scale access to information and services, and provide prevention services to those most at risk, allowing them to adopt safer behaviour.
http://www.ahrn.net/library_upload/uploadfile/file 1844.pdf (accessed October 2005)

159 Sexual and reproductive health and rights: a cornerstone of development. SIDA's contribution to a Swedish policy
Stockholm, Swedish International Development Cooperation Agency (SIDA), 2005. 12 p.

In this paper, the Swedish International Development Co-operation Agency (SIDA) sets out its policy on sexual and reproductive health and rights (SRHR). Sexual and reproductive health is looked at from the perspective of human rights and of the poor, emphasizing the need to address power structures and their impacts. SIDA states its support for culturally sensitive, youth-friendly services, and sexuality and sex education programmes aimed at eliminating prejudice and discrimination for reasons of sex, sexual orientation, gender identity, age or ethnic background. It also advocates integration of SRHR with HIV and AIDS programmes, and the introduction of public financing systems to ensure equal access to high quality sexual and reproductive health care for all. SIDA's priorities in SRHR include contraception, safe abortion, HIV and AIDS and sexually transmitted infections, sexual violence and abuse, harmful traditional practices, and maternal and newborn health. Key strategies include working with the education sector and the field of legislation, and incorporating a gender perspective into all cooperation.
http://www.eldis.org/fulltext/sida-srhr.pdf (accessed October 2005)

160 Sexual and reproductive health (part B4).
Health care services and systems (part B)
In: Global Health Watch 2005-2006. London, Medact, Global Health Watch Secretariat, 2005. 13 p.
The UN International Conference on Population and Development (Cairo, 1994) marked a shift to a broader approach to reproductive health. With the support of UN agencies, the global reproductive health and rights movement has established a women-centred and rights-based framework for action, linking public health, gender equality and development policy. On the other hand, macroeconomic conditions work against the Cairo agenda, and politico-religious fundamentalist approaches undermine the rights agenda and have a negative impact on women. Health activists need to understand the effects of the macroeconomic environment on women's autonomy, sexual and reproductive rights and health. Recommendations for effective change require the human rights framework to be strengthened, alliances to work for economic and social justice, and NGOs and governments to fight against fundamentalisms. Policies for greater bodily integrity should be aligned with social justice and human rights. It is also important to hold donors, governments and institutions accountable, to measure progress on health goals and to produce better research.
http://www.ghwatch.org/2005report/B4.pdf (accessed October 2005)

161 Sexual and reproductive health and rights in the European Union (EU): present status and potential directions for advancement
Warsaw, Federation for Women and Family Planning, Secretariat ASTRA Network, 2004. 13 p.
The situation of women in East Central Europe is markedly different to those in Western Europe. In the east, rates of use of contraception are among the lowest in the world, and abortion is used extensively to control fertility. In the Netherlands, by contrast, where the laws on abortion are very liberal, abortion rates are among the world's lowest. Sexually-transmitted infections including HIV/AIDS are growing fast in the east, with the highest rates among adolescents, whereas HIV/AIDS infections have risen only slightly in western European countries, and antiretroviral treatment has led to lower morbidity and mortality. The EU has the authority to and must ensure that all of its citizens are able to enjoy sexual and reproductive health and rights (SRHR). There are three ways in which SRHR can be promoted: as a human rights issues, as a public health issue, and as an equality issue. The objectives and policies of a number of institutions can be used to advance SRHR throughout the EU.
http://www.astra.org.pl/eu_report.htm (accessed October 2005)

162 Sexual and reproductive health for HIV-positive women: literature review/annotated bibliography
SHIRE, AMY. Joint EngenderHealth/UNFPA project 'HIV prevention in maternal health services and sexual and reproductive health for HIV positive women', 2004. 40 p.
It is only recently that the needs of HIV-infected women have been considered apart from their children, with the result that resource materials and programmes related to the SRH (sexual and reproductive health) needs of HIV-positive women is scarce. Yet the needs are great, ranging from safe contraceptive methods to family planning counseling, as well as health services such as cervical cancer screening. This annotated bibliography of materials on the subject of HIV-positive women is organized around: HIV-positive women's experiences and needs; human rights, stigma and discrimination; SRH services: policies and programme implementation; clinical care and treatment; pregnancy-related decision making, and guidelines and tools. Each of the topics (except the guidelines and tools) is introduced with a summary of overall findings and a description of the sources reviewed. Each section is followed by a list of gaps and emerging issues, and a

concluding resources and materials sections provides background sources on HIV in the context of gender.
http://66.147.176.110/fileadmin/template/main/graphics/eforum/lit_review.pdf (accessed October 2005)

163 Adding it up: the benefits of investing in sexual and reproductive health care
SINGH, SUSHEELA; DARROCH, JACQUELINE E.; VLASSOFF, MICHAEL; NADEAU, JENNIFER. New York, NY, Alan Guttmacher Institute (AGI) with United Nations Population Fund (UNFPA), 2003. 36 p. ISBN 0-939623-62-3
The benefits of sexual and reproductive health care are both medical and non-medical, and have broad social impacts. Policy makers need effective tools to measure the costs and benefits of various health interventions, while taking their broader contributions to society into account. Three major areas are examined: contraceptive services; maternal health services, including prenatal care, obstetric services, postpartum care and abortion-related services; and the prevention, diagnosis and treatment of sexually transmitted infections (STIs), including HIV/AIDS, and other gynaecologic and urologic health care.
http://www.unfpa.org/upload/lib_pub_file/240_filename_addingitup.pdf (accessed October 2005)
KIT Library shelf mark: Br U 04-13

164 Enhancing gender equity in health programmes: monitoring and evaluation
SMITH, MOHGA KAMAL. *Gender and Development* 9(2001)2, p. 95-105 ISSN 1355-2074
Gender-sensitive monitoring and evaluating in health programmes ensures that interventions improve public health, positively influence women and relations between men and women, and help to reduce poverty. A lack of sensitivity to gender may mean programmes fail and even worsen women's position in the home or in the community. The aim of monitoring is to highlight what changes in policy or practices may be needed to achieve programme goals. Evaluation of programmes assesses the degree of achievement of stated objectives. Monitoring the impact of user fees, for example, illustrates the effect of gender identity on access to medical care. Successful gender-sensitive monitoring and evaluation requires sufficient human and financial resources to function, and the commitment of organizations to build the capacity of health professionals for planning and implementation.
KIT Library shelf mark: D 3030-9(2001)2

165 Towards reproductive health for all?
STANDING, HILARY. In: Targeting development: critical perspectives on the Millennium Development Goals ed. by Richard Black and Howard White. London, Routledge, 2004, p. 235-255
The Programme of Action established through the International Conference on Population and Development (ICPD) and the Millennium Development Goals (MDGs) differ, due to a continuing political struggle over women's rights to sexual and reproductive health services. The reduction of maternal mortality is a target in its own right in the MDGs, but family planning is only an indicator for monitoring the HIV/AIDS targets. The broader aim of the ICPD needs to be retained while respecting different levels of developmental capacity. The specific MDGs on maternal health emphasizing the reduction of maternal mortality can only be achieved within the broader commitment to reproductive health.
KIT Library shelf mark: N 04-498

166 Synergising HIV/AIDS and sexual and reproductive health and rights: a manual for NGOs
Copenhagen, AIDSNET, the Danish NGO Network on AIDS and Development, 2005. 63 p.
The manual deals with the arguments and rationale behind integrating HIV/AIDS and sexual and reproductive health and rights (SRHR). It emphasizes important societal aspects of the framework for integrated HIV/AIDS and SRHR activities, discusses the most important health system factors, and addresses how NGO's can integrate HIV/AIDS and SSRHR.
http://www.aidsnet.dk/files/filer/aidsnet/sm/extranet/srhr%20manual/aidsnetwhosynergisingmanualfinal.pdf (accessed October 2005)

167 Cutting edge pack: gender and HIV/AIDS
TALLIS, V.; BELL, E. Brighton, Briefings on Gender and Development (BRIDGE), University of Sussex, 2002
This pack contains three documents which address issues of gender inequality and HIV/AIDS. The overview report utilizes a gendered human rights framework and advocates for ensuing policy and programmes on HIV/AIDS are informed by the complex and diverse realities of women, men and children's lives. The resources document includes summaries of resources, case studies, summaries on toolkits and guides, information on websites. The third document contains short articles on gender and HIV/AIDS projects and other activities.
http://www.bridge.ids.ac.uk/reports_gend_CEP.html#HIV (accessed October 2005)

168 'Sector-wide approaches: opportunities and challenges for gender equity in health'. Papers presented at Women's World Conference, Kampala, Uganda, 23rd and 24th July 2002
THEOBALD, SALLY; TOLHURST, RACHEL; ELSEY, HELEN (eds). Liverpool, Gender and Health Group, Liverpool School of Tropical Medicine (LSTM), 2002. refs. 159 p.
Sector-wide approaches (SWAps) are aid programmes in which donors contribute to development within the framework of a locally-owned strategy and approach. Major themes under discussion relating to gender mainstreaming in SWAps are how to create a facilitative environment, the involvement of different stakeholder interests, and facilitation through instruments and processes. Gender mainstreaming requires building alliances, developing consensus and momentum. CSOs/NGOs, government and development partners must learn to work together and build trust, towards the creation of more positive and equal partnerships. The pace of change is likely to be slow in developing initiatives for gender equity. It is helpful to develop synergies between gender training and other training needs. An increase of gender awareness among facilitators of participatory processes will also ensure that women's voices are heard. Stronger gender-equitable participation in health service provision could involve greater community participation in data collection and use, and in identifying meaningful participation opportunities.
http://www.liv.ac.uk/lstm/research/documents/Resource_pack.pdf (accessed October 2005)

169 Gender, health and development I: gender equity and sector wide approaches
THEOBALD, SALLY; ELSEY; HELEN; TOLHURST, RACHEL. *Progress in Development Studies* 4(2004)1, p. 58-63 ISSN 1464-9934
There has been growth in the number of sector wide approaches (SWAps) in Asia and especially Africa in the health, education and transport sectors. Their aim is to improve coordination and benefits and build capacity for sustained, effective policies and programmes. While gender equity is not the central focus of SWAps, there are synergies between them and initiatives with explicit equity goals such as the Poverty Reduction Strategy. However, the synergies may be more theoretical than practical as yet. The report presented here is based on the results of a workshop to examine gender mainstreaming in SWAps in eight different countries including Uganda, Ghana, Ethiopia and Bangladesh. The donor-driven nature of SWAps could be a potential hazard, especially where public participation and local gender activism within government ministries is limited. Additionally, very few SWAps (4 out of about 80 worldwide) have government support. While SWAps offer new opportunities and challenges, gender advocates need new skills and strategies to help bring about gender mainstreaming. The workshop identified a need for training and awareness-raising.
KIT Library shelf mark: H 2859-4(2004)1

170 Gender, health and development (II): gender equity and access to antiretroviral drugs
THEOBALD, SALLY; TAEGTMEYER, MIRIAM. *Progress in Development Studies* 5(2005)2, p. 144-148 ISSN 1464-9934
Antiretroviral drugs (ARVs) have radically reduced mortality and in-patient rates and improved the quality of life of HIV patients in the west during the last decade. Of the majority of people with HIV/AIDS, however, an average of only 5% of the estimated 5.5 million adults in resource-poor regions needing ARVs appear to have access to them. In spite of stated global political commitment to large-scale availability of drugs, it will be impossible to provide access to ARVs to everyone who needs them in the near future. While there is little published information on which sectors of the population are accessing ARVs for HIV prevention or treatment, some estimates indicate probable gender inequities in access and use. More, relatively wealthier men use ARVs in spite of the 1:1.5 ratio of men to women reportedly infected in some areas, e.g. sub-Saharan Africa. In Thika District, Kenya, 71% of HIV clinic clients are women, but only 48% of the clients on ARVs are women, for reasons of lack of money for drugs or even transport to clinics. Links between gender and poverty are also indicated in Uganda, when there is insufficient money for both husband and wife to have ARVs. Inequitable delivery and access to ARVs is tied to inequitable health policies and practices. Further debate and shared lessons from other health care programmes are needed to promote gender and equity, particularly in view of women's and girl's greater vulnerability to HIV infection.
KIT Library shelf mark: H 2859-5(2005)2

171 Teaching about gender, health, and communicable disease: experiences and challenges
TOLHURST, RACHEL; THEOBALD, SALLY. *Gender and Development* 9(2001)2, p. 74-86 ISSN 1355-2074
There is a perceived lack of awareness among development policy makers and planners as to

the links between gender, health and infectious diseases. Gender training requires group work and reflection on the personal, as well as professional, experiences of participants. Participants in the course on gender and health learned how mainstreaming gender into the work and structure of health institutions is important. It is shown to influence health interventions, e.g. in terms of priority setting. A SWOT (strengths-weaknesses-opportunities-threats) analysis helps to identify the implications of gender-sensitive planning within institutions. Student feedback from the course helps to guide future directions and course content; and the development of skills and responses relevant to course participants' working situations.

172 Women of the world: laws and policies affecting their reproductive lives: South Asia
UPRETI, MELISSA. New York, NY, Center for Reproductive Lives, 2004. 242 p. ISBN 1-890671-10-X
The report presents an examination of laws and policies that influence women's reproductive health in five countries of the region: Bangladesh, India, Nepal, Pakistan and Sri Lanka. The report, which is based on three years of research, is the result of a collaborative partnership between the Center and leading NGOs in the region. It offers advocates and policy makers a broad view of the laws and policies that determine women's reproductive choices in these countries, to enable legal and policy reform and the implementation of norms needed to improve women's health and lives. The report is a resource for those interested in advancing and protecting women's reproductive health and rights through legal advocacy and establishing state accountability for violations of reproductive rights.
http://www.reproductiverights.org/pub_bo_wowsa.html#toc

173 Violence against women: the health sector responds
VELZEBOER, MARIJKE; ELLSBERG, MARY; CLAVEL ARCAS, CARMEN; GARCIA-MORENO, CLAUDIA. *Occasional Publication* 12. Washington, DC, Pan American Health Organization (PAHO), 2003. 131 p. refs. ISBN 92-75-12292-X
There are opportunities for the health sector to help prevent gender-based violence. Obviously, no one model of effective intervention fits all, and different contexts must always be taken into account. However, many lessons learned from specific experiences in Central America can be applied elsewhere. The approach used by PAHO

is based on Critical Path Studies. The approach is flexible and non-prescriptive, with no drive to impose a general model on all settings. It calls for action at several levels: national, public and community. A multi-sectoral approach achieves the best results, when a dynamic is achieved between health, education and law enforcement. Partnerships and networks are needed to provide a platform to support women living with violence.

174 The role of men in the fight against HIV/AIDS
WAINAINA, NJOKI. Paper presented at the Expert Group Meeting on 'The role of men and boys in achieving gender equality', 21-24 October 2003, Brasilia, Brazil. *EGM/Men-Boys-GE/2003/EP.4*. Geneva, United Nations, 2003. 11 p.
Equality is a human rights issue. Building partnerships between men and women addresses one of the root causes of the spread of HIV/AIDS: unequal gender power relations. Increasingly, men are mobilizing against gender-based violence and the fight against HIV/AIDS, for example with the Men for Gender Equality Initiative in Africa. Men are beginning to see the need to construct new masculinities that promote gender equality. Countries like Uganda and Kenya offer lessons on how to mobilize and involve men through schools, faith-based groups, labour groups and communities. Programmes should communicate with people in ways that are consistent with local cultures and include all members of society, rather than targeting high-risk groups. Men should be involved in educational programmes and in designing interventions to reach other men. Hope for the future lies in changing the attitudes and behaviour of boys, men of tomorrow who will not be afraid of gender equality.
http://www.un.org/womenwatch/daw/egm/men-boys2003/EP4-Wainaina.pdf (accessed October 2005)

175 What's sex and gender got to do with it? Integrating sex and gender into health research. Final report of the first International think tank on Sex, Gender and Health, February 27-March 1, 2003
Edmonton, Institute of Gender and Health (IGH), 2004
Participants in the Institute of Gender and Health (IGH) think tank agree that sex and gender require greater attention in health research. Sex and gender cannot simply be equated with biology and culture; they are influenced by race and ethnicity, socioeconomics, sexual identity and orientation, politics and

history. Innovative methods and tools are needed to understand their significance for health research. The IGH can continue to deepen understanding of sex and gender in relation to health by promoting the creation of new frameworks, identifying existing tools, supporting the creation of new analytical instruments, and by launching initiatives addressing the concerns of Aboriginal women, men and children.

http://www.cihr-irsc.gc.ca/e/25131.html (accessed October 2005)

176 Men and reproductive health programs: influencing gender norms
WHITE, VICTORIA; GREENE, MARGARET; MURPHY, ELAINE. The Synergy Project. USAID, 2003. 64 p.
Gender roles affect HIV/AIDS as well as reproductive, maternal and child health. Raising awareness of the influences of gender norms and behaviours can give programmes addressing these reproductive health issues a positive direction. It is important to involve men in efforts to alter social norms towards equality of resources and rights. for women. Various programmes are based on the Diffusion of Innovations theory by Everett Rogers. The theory describes a process whereby early adopters of new behaviours tend to be peer group leaders. Only when a critical mass of adopters develops, is it possible for society and social norms to change. While numerous programmes designed to change gender norms have been carried out, few have been evaluated in a way that would make them replicable. Several are nevertheless recognized as innovative and influential, e.g., Fathers Inc. in Jamaica, PAPAI in Brazil, CORAIC and Salud y Género in Mexico, and others in the Himalayas, the Dominican Republic, Botswana, Zambia and Kenya. Good programmes can accelerate the pace of progress. The evaluated programmes were specifically designed to address social norms related to gender roles, explaining the methods used and presenting findings from various evaluations of their efficacy.

http://www.synergyaids.com/SynergyPublications/Gender_Norms.pdf (accessed October 2005)

177 WHO gender policy: integrating gender perspectives in the work of WHO
Geneva, World Health Organization (WHO), 2002. 6 p.
The WHO gender policy for the integration of gender perspectives sets out the background and rationale, goal and objectives, and organizational arrangements for implementation. It contains a 'gender glossary' explaining how gender is understand in terms of analysis, equality, equity and mainstreaming. Since gender is an issue with widespread implications in many different contexts, the gender policy is important for every staff member of WHO. The organization's commitment to the integration of gender perspectives should be reflected in work plans and budgets as well as activities in cooperation with countries. Action plans for the inclusion of gender perspectives developed by various departments and offices are used to monitor the progress of integration.

http://www.who.int/gender/documents/en/engpolicy.pdf (accessed October 2005)

178 Women and health (including HIV and human rights): findings of the online discussion
In: Summary of the online discussions held in preparation for the 10 year review and appraisal of the implementation of the Platform for Action in the 49th session of the Commission on the Status of Women. New York, NY, Inter-Agency Network on Women and Gender Equality (IANWGE), 2005. p. 15-30
The Joint United Nations Programme on HIV/AIDS (UNAIDS), the World Health Organization (WHO), and the United Nations Population Fund (UNFPA) organized the online discussion on Women and Health in three phases from 10 November 2004 to 24 January 2005. The Moderator was Subidita Chatterjee. The discussion was organized in three phases: general and health systems issues (including communicable and non-communicable diseases); sexual and reproductive health (including HIV and human rights); and rights, needs and support for HIV-positive women and girls and those vulnerable to the virus. There were 601 participants in all, from national machineries for the advancement of women, United Nations entities, faith-based organizations and women's groups. They included women activists; academics; policy makers; gender equality researchers and practitioners; health-care providers; people living with HIV/AIDS, and other members of the international community. A summary of outcomes is presented.

http://www.un.org/womenwatch/forums/review/IANWGEOnlineDiscussionReport.pdf (accessed October 2005)

179 Women and health: new challenges. Beijing at 10: putting policy into practice
Santo Domingo, United Nations International Research and Training Institute for the Advancement of Women (UN INSTRAW), 2005. 19 p.

The Beijing Platform of Action and Programme of Action of the International Conference on Population and Development are the only international instruments that take a broad perspective on women's health, going beyond maternal health issues to addresses the impact of gender throughout the life cycle. This review appraises developments since Beijing, looking at implementation of actions towards four strategic objectives identified within critical area C: Women and Health, specifically relating to women's access to health services, preventive programmes to promote women's health, gender-sensitive initiatives addressing sexual and reproductive health issues and HIV/AIDS, information dissemination and research, and increased resources and monitoring. Overall, goals set for 2015 would appear to be unachievable, due to the inadequate or non-existent implementation of many recommendations. Public health systems worldwide are deteriorating and disappearing following public sector reforms and privatization. Gender inequality continues to threaten women's health, since it means lack of access to health services and information and exposure to abuse, HIV infection and unwanted pregnancy. The review identifies areas for future action in each of the strategic sub-sections, and calls for more gender-specific research as well as the inclusion of women in health decision making processes.
http://www.un-instraw.org/en/images/stories/Beijing/womenandhealth.pdf (accessed October 2005)

180 Women and HIV/AIDS: confronting the crisis
ERB-LEONCAVALLO, ANN; HOLMES, GILLIAN; JACOBS, GLORIA; MICOL, ZARB; URDANG, STEPHANIE; VANEK, JOANN. Geneva, UNAIDS/UNFPA/UNIFEM, 2004. 76 p.
The report examines the current situation from the perspectives of prevention, treatment, care-giving, education, violence and women's rights. In conclusion, recommendations are offered for charting the way forward.
http://www.unfpa.org/upload/lib_pub_file/308_filename_women_aids1.pdf (accessed October 2005)

181 Women's mental health: an evidence based review
ASTBURY, JILL; CABRAL, MEENA. WHO/MSD/MDP/00.1. Geneva, Department of Mental Health and Substance Dependence, World Health Organization (WHO), 2000. 122 p.
Depression is thought to become the second most important cause of disease in the world by 2020, and women are almost twice as likely as men to experience it. Other leading causes of the disease burden, violence and self-inflicted injuries, are also considered to be relevant to women's mental health. Social and cultural inequalities between men and women are contributory risk factors for women's mental health, as illustrated in the significantly different rates of depression between men and women, the impact of poverty, and violence against women. The evidence reviewed covers socio-economic factors in gender development and health, social theories of depression, the relationships between poverty, social position and mental health and various aspects of violence against women in different contexts. Analysis of this evidence is intended to provide guidance for research and action.
http://whqlibdoc.who.int/hq/2000/WHO_MSD_MDP_00.1.pdf (accessed October 2005)

182 Sexual and reproductive health: a foundation for achieving the MDGs
WOODS, ZONIBEL. Paper prepared for the United Nations Division for the Advancement of Women (DAW) Expert Group meeting 'Achievements, Gaps and Challenges in Linking the Implementation of The Beijing Platform for Action and the Millennium Declaration and Millennium Development Goals', Baku, Azerbaijan, 7-10 February 2005. *EGM/BPFA-MD-MDG/2005/EP.9*. Geneva, United Nations, 2005. 12 p.
Progress in the areas of education for girls and access to contraception for women has been made since the early 1990s. However, the relationship between gender equality and reproductive health and rights is not always sufficiently understood. A third of illnesses and early deaths among women aged 15-49 is still related to reproductive and sexual problems. 62% of people aged 15-24 living with HIV/AIDS worldwide are young women. In many countries, being a married women is a high risk factor. Gender is also a factor in the spread, impact and treatment of HIV/AIDS. Responses to the situation should include reproductive health services, the promotion of education for girls, changes in property rights and economic opportunities for women, open discussion about sexuality, gender, safe sex, and the need to change traditional norms. Important areas that require attention are women's rights to control their sexuality, the right of adolescents to sexual and reproductive health services and education, and abortion laws. The Millennium Project Taskforce 4 Report states that adolescents deserve special attention. With so many (1 billion) now making the transition from childhood to adulthood, they are key if the Millennium Goals are to be met in a sustainable way. Recommendations for action include giving

urgent attention to providing safe abortion, reviewing laws and practices that jeopardize women's health, sex education, and ensuring universal access to sexual and reproductive health services as part of the response to AIDS.
http://www.un.org/womenwatch/daw/egm/bpfamd2005/experts-papers/EGM-BPFA-MD-MDG-2005-EP.9.pdf (accessed October 2005)

183 Working from within: culturally sensitive approaches in UNFPA programming
New York, United Nations Population Fund (UNFPA), 2004. 36 p.
Issues surrounding reproductive health and rights are intimate and sensitive, making it important to find acceptable ways of working with people towards improvement. Outsiders may find it difficult to understand age-old traditions and patterns that surround people's lives in different cultures. They present challenges, but also opportunities for development. Some of these are described in nine case studies of culturally-sensitive United Nations Population Fund (UNFPA) initiatives around the world, with indications of what works or what could work. Culturally-sensitive approaches facilitate programme implementation because they create a positive negotiation environment through understanding. They acknowledge the need for patience and transparency, and respect people's culture and its expressions while promoting universally-recognized human rights. Facilitating an environment in which principles of human rights and gender equity can be established helps people to appreciate the principles and incorporate them into their own reality. Partnering with local cultural and religious leaders is important to help defuse potential tension and focus on the goal of improving people's well being. Where advocacy campaigns are developed, they more effectively reach a wide audience when they are closely matched to the appropriate cultural context, and draw on popular sources. Music, poetry and drama is used in Uganda, for example, and in Muslim contexts, the use of Islamic references can help to promote local ownership.
http://www.unfpa.org/upload/lib_pub_file/268_filename_Culture_2004.pdf (accessed October 2005)

184 Working with men, responding to AIDS. Gender, sexuality and HIV: a case study collection
Brighton, International HIV/AIDS Alliance, 2003. 68 p.
The International HIV/AIDS Alliance and its partners in Africa, Asia, Eastern Europe and Latin America are increasingly focusing on the roles and responsibilities of men in the community response to HIV/AIDS. This has involved identifying what their roles and responsibilities are in different contexts, and developing strategies to work with men on them. This case study collection is produced to help projects to conduct this work with men on HIV/AIDS. It presents experiences and lessons in the form of case studies from a range of different projects that are working with men, and thereby aims to offer ideas and models for working with different kinds of men in a range of contexts.
http://www.aidsalliance.org/graphics/secretariat/publications/wwm1103_working_with_men.pdf (accessed October 2005)

185 The World Health Report 2005: Make every mother and child count. Overview
MANUEL, ANNICK; MATTHEWS, ZOË; VAN LERBERGHE, WIM; WOLFHEIM, CATHY.
Geneva, World Health Organization (WHO), 2005. 16 p.
The Millennium Development Goals highlighted the importance of mother and child health as an integral part of poverty reduction. Progress towards achieving the goals has been erratic, but accelerated improvements are possible towards achieve the goals by the target date of 2015. A renewed focus of maternal and child health is needed, with an emphasis on newborns. Millions of babies die each year, 3.3 million of them stillborn and another 4 million within 28 days of birth. In some countries, maternal, newborn and child health (MNCH) indicators have stagnated in recent years, or even reversed. The technical knowledge exists to respond to the situation, and placing the emphasis on MNCH provides a platform for sustainable health systems. Effective antenatal care can be used as a platform for HIV/AIDS and STI prevention, and other health interventions. MNCH programmes are most effective if they provide a continuum of care from pregnancy into childhood, as part of the broader context of health system development. The ultimate goal is to provide universal access to health care systems.
http://www.who.int/whr/2005/overview_en.pdf (accessed October 2005)

186 Young men and HIV prevention
BARKER, GARY; HUTCHINSON, SHERRY; PULERWITZ, JULIE; SEGUNDO, MARCIO; WEISS, ELLEN. In: *Horizons Report* (2004)December. New York, NY, Population Council, 2004. 12 p.
Progress on slowing the AIDS epidemic among women and girls cannot be accomplished without programmes that address gender inequality, and

which also involve men and boys. Gender norms are an important factor, particularly among the young. Unequal power relationships can lead to sexual violence, and inequity can also serious affect men. 'Traditional' ideas of manhood, for example, can lead to increased drug use, violence and unsafe sex. Group interventions in Brazil found associations between gender norms and HIV risk variables. Gender-based interventions for young men can reduce their level of HIV risk. In Tanzania, research shows how gender roles limit communication, because of lack of trust between men and women. Current interventions focus on encouraging fidelity and greater respect, trust and improved communication between the sexes. Knowledge about HIV/AIDS is low in India, yet 4.6 million are infected with HIV. Group programmes address gender, masculinity and sexuality, gender-based violence and HIV/AIDS. Initial results show a high level of participation among the target group.
http://www.popcouncil.org/pdfs/horizons/hrptdec04.pdf (accessed October 2005)

187 The gender guide for health communication programs
ZAMAN, FARIA; UNDERWOOD, CAROL. Baltimore, Johns Hopkins Bloomberg School of Public Health/Center for Communication Programs, Population Communication Services, 2003. 28 p.
The guide contains contributions by individuals and organizations committed to gender equity, including members of the USAID/Interagency Gender Working Group, health communications in Nepal and Ghana and in Asia, Africa, Latin America and the Near East. The guide supports the inclusion of gender-based roles and responsibilities in health communication programmes. While it does not directly address issues of gender equity, it provides questions to enable programme managers to identify relevant information on the access to, use and limitations of health services. The questions promote dialogue in communities with the intention of increasing understanding of gender issues. The information obtained can be used to encourage attention being given to resolving inequities. The guide is intended for professionals involved in the development of health communication programmes. It is easy to use, following the consecutive steps of development of a communication programme: analysis, strategic design, message/materials development, pre-testing and production, management, implementation and monitoring, and evaluation.

It is flexible, with each step suitable for use independently of other steps.
http://www.jhuccp.org/pubs/cp/102/102.pdf (accessed October 2005)

188 Gender, sexuality and the criminal laws in the Middle East and North Africa: a comparative study
ZUHUR, SHERIFA. Istanbul, Women for Women's Human Rights (WWHR) – New Ways, 2005. refs. 76 p.
Reforms in family law in the Middle East and North Africa and the Muslim world are not enough to overcome human rights violations and discrimination against women; penal or criminal codes also require reform. The study examines laws in the region relating to issues of honour, murder and adultery, rape, incest and sexual abuse, illegitimacy and abortion, reproductive technologies, sex work and trafficking in women, and female genital mutilation. This survey shows that some laws have changed over time. Others are yet to be adjusted to meet the demands of today.
http://www.wwhr.org/images/GenderSexualityand CriminalLaws.pdf (accessed October 2005)

Author index

(numbers refer to abstract numbers)

author index

167

Subject index

Geographical Index

(numbers refer to abstract numbers)

Web resources

Female genital mutilation

Female Genital Cutting (FGC) Education and Networking Project
The purpose of the FGC Education and Networking Project is the online and offline dissemination of material related to female genital mutilation (FGM). The Project provides an online clearinghouse and community for researchers, activists, attorneys, and health care practitioners to obtain information and network with others involved in similar projects. The site provides access to relevant information sources on Africa and the Middle East, on national US and international legislation, and on international eradication efforts.
http://www.fgmnetwork.org/html/index.php (accessed January 2006)

Foundation for Women's Health Research and Development (FORWARD)
FORWARD is an international NGO dedicated to improving the health and well being of African women and girls, wherever they reside. FORWARD promotes action to stop harmful traditional practices, such as FGM and early and forced marriages, which violate the human rights of women and girls and adversely affect their health and well being. The site provides information about where to find help and advice, and training; a list of FGM publications; a video library; and links to FGM sites.
http://www.forwarduk.org.uk/ (accessed January 2006)

INTACT Network
The International Network to Analyze, Communicate and Transform the Campaign against Female Genital Cutting (INTACT) aims to promote and disseminate evidence-based research and to actively engage donors and local actors, governments and civil society organizations in a dialogue around applying collective learning to accelerate positive social change. The website contains information on the network's activities, research, publications and a forum for the exchange of information and discussion.
http://www.intact-network.net/ (last accessed January 2006)

The Research Action and Information Network for the Bodily Integrity of Women (RAINBO)
RAINBO is an African led international NGO working on women's empowerment, gender, reproductive health, sexual autonomy and freedom from violence. The organization specifically strives to enhance global efforts to eliminate the practice of FGM by facilitating women's self-empowerment and accelerating social change. The website offers access to information on their work, the small grants project and the African immigrant programme, and their publications.
http://www.rainbo.org (last accessed January 2006)

Tostan, Women's Health and Human Rights
Tostan, an international NGO based in Senegal, combines traditional and modern techniques to help bring about positive change on the personal, community and national level. This model of education has been used as a strategy for ending FGM in Senegal and Burkina Faso. Information on Tostan's activities, articles and links is presented.
http://www.tostan.org (last accessed January 2006)

Health

The Asian-Pacific Resource & Research Centre for Women (ARROW)
ARROW is committed to promoting and protecting women's health rights and needs, particularly in the area of women's sexuality and reproductive health, in Asia and the Pacific. Its information and documentation centre houses a collection of over 10 000 titles, including

web resources

published and unpublished materials on women and health.
http://www.arrow.org.my (last accessed January 2006)

Centre for Health and Gender Equity (CHANGE)
CHANGE is a US-based NGO that focuses on the effects of US international policies on the health and rights of women, girls, and other vulnerable populations in Africa, Asia, and Latin America.
http://www.genderhealth.org/ (last accessed January 2006)

Engender Health
Engender Health works in over 30 countries, specializing in some key health issues for women and their families. It provides family planning training, innovative safe-motherhood programmes, partnerships to transform care, services for men, and quality-improvement programmes.
http://www.engenderhealth.org (last accessed January 2006)

Equality Now
Equality Now works to end violence and discrimination against women through the mobilization of public pressure. Issues of concern include: reproductive rights, FGM, and domestic violence.
http://www.equalitynow.org/ (last accessed January 2006)

Gender and Health Equity Network
The Network is a partnership of national and international institutions concerned with developing and implementing policies to improve gender and health equity, particularly in resource constrained environments. The website includes summaries of the country case studies, together with resources on gender and health equity.
http://www.ids.ac.uk/ghen/ (last accessed January 2006)

Gender, Ethnicity and Health Unit, Pan American Health Organization (PAHO)
The mandate of the Gender, Ethnicity and Health Unit is to integrate a gender and ethnic perspective into PAHO's projects, programmes and policies. Information is one of the tools used to do this. The website provides information on the following subjects: violence against women; health policies; and gender mainstreaming. It also offers access to the GenSalud Information System that provides information on the effects of gender on the health of women and men in the Americas.
http://www.paho.org/English/ad/ge/home.htm (last accessed January 2006)

Gender, Women and Health (GWH) Department, World Health Organization (WHO)
GWH brings attention to the ways in which biological and social differences between women and men affect health, and the steps needed to achieve health equity. The main focus is to promote the inclusion of gender perspectives in the work of the WHO by collaborating with other departments and regional and country offices. Information and publications on various gender and health topics are presented.
http://www.who.int/gender/en/ (last accessed January 2006)

Instituto Promundo
Instituto Promundo is a Brazilian NGO that works internationally to promote gender equality and child and youth development. It carries out programme development and research, and provides technical assistance related to the socialization of young men and women, health promotion, HIV/AIDS prevention, respect for sexual diversity and violence prevention in Latin America, Asia and sub-Saharan Africa. The website contains information on their programmes, research and campaigns, and provides access to support materials.
http://www.promundo.org.br (last accessed January 2006)

10th International Women and Health meeting 'Health Rights, Women's Lives: Challenges and Strategies for Movement Building'
This website contains information on the 10th International Women and Health meeting, New Delhi, India, which was held on 21-25 September 2005. It includes information on the five focal themes that have been addressed at the meeting and provides access to an online book of abstracts of papers.
http://www.10iwhmindia.org/ (last accessed January 2006)

International Centre for Research on Women (ICRW)
ICRW is a private, non-profit organization dedicated to improving the lives of women in poverty, advancing equality and human rights, and contributing to broader economic and social well being. ICRW's research, technical support and advocacy work focuses on adolescence, HIV/AIDS, nutrition & food security, poverty reduction, reproductive health & population, violence against women, and women's rights. The website provides access to information on

ICRW's work by issue, by project and by publication.
http://www.icrw.org/ (last accessed January 2006)

The Key Centre for Women's Health in Society
The Key Centre for Women's Health in Society, School of Population Health, University of Melbourne, Australia, has been at the forefront of thinking, researching, teaching and information dissemination about women's health.
http://www.kcwh.unimelb.edu.au (last accessed January 2006)

Latin American and Caribbean Women's Health Network (LACWHN)
LACWHN is a network of organizations and individuals that aims to be a political reference point within the women's health movement and the wider society in order to: influence national and international public policies; to monitor these policy processes as part of civil society; and generate and disseminate relevant knowledge. The website presents their research, training, advocacy and promotion activities, and their publications, including the Women's Health Journal.
http://www.reddesalud.org/ (last accessed January 2006)

Programme for Appropriate Technology (PATH)
PATH is an international organization whose mission is to improve health, especially the health of women and children.
http://www.path.org (last accessed January 2006)

Women and Health Programme, World Health Organization Centre for Health Development (WHO Kobe Centre)
The Women and Health Programme (WHP) was created in 2000 to address issues related to women's health and welfare through research. The research programme was designed to facilitate the identification, collection, analysis and dissemination of up-to-date information on effective policies, programmes and strategies that could contribute to the improvement of the health and welfare of women and their families. At its Third International Meeting on Women and Health (2002), WHP issued the Kobe Plan of Action for Women and Health and used it as a framework to identify its research priorities. Information on research activities and programmes, as well as meeting reports and publications, are presented on the website.
http://www.who.or.jp/WHP/index.html (last accessed January 2006)

Women's Health Project (WHP)
WHP, a project of the Witwatersrand University, South Africa, is concerned with research, training and advocacy. The website provides information on campaigns, publications and training in the field of reproductive rights & health, sexual rights, health system transformation, and gender.
http://www.wits.ac.za/whp/ (last accessed January 2006)

HIV/AIDS

Gender-AIDS Forum
Gender-AIDS is an international e-forum that facilitates linkages and information sharing between people living with HIV/AIDS groups, women's organizations and other organizations working or interested in the area of gender and HIV/AIDS. Gender-AIDS is coordinated by the Health & Development Networks eForum Resource Team (HDN, www.hdnet.org) with the support of Development Cooperation Ireland (DCI, www.dci.gov.ie).
To join, send a blank message to **join-gender-aids@eforums.healthdev.org**

Gender and HIV/AIDS, UNAIDS
This website includes key documents and resources on gender and HIV/AIDS.
http://www.unaids.org/Unaids/EN/In+focus/Topic+areas/Women_gender.asp (last accessed January 2006)

Gender and HIV/AIDS web portal, UNIFEM
UNIFEM in collaboration with UNAIDS has developed this gender and HIV/AIDS web portal to provide up-to-date information on the gender dimensions of the HIV/AIDS epidemic. The web portal provides access to a variety of materials such as cutting edge research, studies and surveys; training materials; multi-media advocacy tools; speeches and presentations; press releases and current news.
http://www.genderandaids.org/ (last accessed January 2006)

Global Coalition on Women and AIDS (GCWA), UNAIDS initiative
GCWA is a worldwide alliance of civil society groups, networks of women with HIV/AIDS, governments and UN organizations. The Coalition works at global, regional and national levels to highlight the impact of AIDS on women and girls and mobilize actions to enable them to protect themselves from HIV and receive the care and support they need. The GCWA was launched by UNAIDS. The website presents

web resources

175

information on regional activities, and information resources such as background briefs, speeches and other publications. http://womenandaids.unaids.org/ (last accessed January 2006)

Safe motherhood

Safe Motherhood
In January 2004, an expanded Partnership for Safe Motherhood and Newborn Health was established with the aim of promoting the health of women and newborns, especially the most vulnerable. The Partnership aims to strengthen maternal and newborn health efforts at the global, regional, and national levels, in the context of equity, poverty reduction, and human rights. The Partnership's priorities, international commitments, and information resources can be accessed through the website. http://www.safemotherhood.org (last accessed January 2006)

Sex work

Network of Sex Work Projects
The Network is an international organization for promoting sex workers' health and human rights. With member organizations in more than 40 countries, the Network develops partnerships with technical support agencies to work on independently-financed projects. The website provides access to resources in the field of health and safety, rights, mobility, ethics, laws and culture all over the world. http://www.nswp.org (last accessed January 2006)

Sex-Work Forum
An international e-forum to facilitate discussion around sex work and HIV/AIDS. Sex-Work is coordinated by the Health & Development Networks eForum Resource Team (HDN, www.hdnet.org) with the support of Development Cooperation Ireland (DCI, www.dci.gov.ie) To join, send a blank message to: join-sex-work@eforums.healthdev.org

Sexual and Reproductive Health and Rights

Alan Guttmacher Institute (AGI)
The US-based AGI focuses on reproductive health research, policy analysis and public education. The information on the website can be accessed by subject: abortion, adolescents, contraception, men, pregnancy, services & financing, sex & relationships, STIs & HIV/AIDS, technology and bioethics. The Institute's periodicals, including Perspectives on Sexual and Reproductive Health, can also be searched or browsed. http://www.agi-usa.org (last accessed January 2006)

Central and Eastern European Women's Network for Sexual and Reproductive Health and Rights (ASTRA Network)
http://www.astra.org.pl/index.php (last accessed January 2006)

The Centre for African Family Studies (CAFS)
CAFS conducts courses and provides research and consultancy services from its headquarters in Nairobi, Kenya and its regional office in Lomé, Togo. It also conducts operations research, community surveys and applied research focusing on the African family. http://www.cafs.org (last accessed January 2006)

Countdown 2015: Sexual and Reproductive Health and Rights for All
This initiative is dedicated to assessing the progress towards the key goals of the International Conference on Population and Development (ICPD), held in Cairo in 1994. It aims to identify future directions, recruit new allies, and recognize the critical role of young people in the efforts to meet the commitments made at ICPD. Countdown 2015 comprises a series of activities and events that will be held throughout 2004 and into 2005, and is a key element of efforts by NGOs and civil society to mark the tenth anniversary of ICPD at the national, regional and international levels. http://www.countdown2015.org/ (last accessed January 2006)

European Non-Governmental Organizations for Sexual and Reproductive Health and Rights, Population and Development (EuroNGOs)
EuroNGOs seek to translate the commitments of the International Conference on Population and Development (ICPD, 1994) into international cooperative programmes in the field of sexual and reproductive health in developing countries. http://www.eurongos.org (last accessed January 2006)

Family Care International (FCI)
FCI is dedicated to improving women's sexual and reproductive health and rights in developing countries, with a special emphasis on making pregnancy and childbirth safer. http://www.familycareintl.org (last accessed January 2006)

Family Health International (FHI)
FHI works to improve reproductive and family health around the world through biomedical and social science research, innovative health service delivery interventions, training and information programmes.
http://www.fhi.org (last accessed January 2006)

Fundación para Estudio e Investigación de la Mujer (FEIM)
FEIM is a foundation for research on women. It focuses on reproductive health and sexual health rights for women and youth. It started its work on HIV/AIDS in 1990. Information on their work and publications, and news and events is presented in Spanish.
http://www.feim.org.ar/ (last accessed January 2006)

Gender and Reproductive Rights, World Health Organization (WHO)
The website includes materials and resources as well as working definitions of sex, sexuality, sexual health, sexual rights. The working definitions were elaborated as a result of a WHO-convened international technical consultation on sexual health in January 2002, and subsequently revised by a group of experts from different parts of the world. The site is part of WHO's Reproductive Health and Research website.
http://www.who.int/reproductive-health/gender/index.html (last accessed January 2006)

Improving Reproductive Health, Swiss Agency for Development and Cooperation (SDC)
Improving reproductive health is one of the priorities in health of the SDC, with a focus on reproductive health and rights, maternal health, FGM (and gender-based violence) and early childhood. The website includes documents and other information resources.
http://www.sdc-health.ch/priorities_in_health/reproductive_health (last accessed January 2006)

The Initiative for Sexual and Reproductive Rights in Health Reforms
This research and advocacy initiative aims to strengthen understanding among activists and decision makers of the role of health sector reform in facilitating or undermining efforts to achieve sexual and reproductive health policies and programmes. Key foci are: health financing, public-private partnership, priority setting in relation to the primary care package, decentralization of services, and integration of services. The website contains information on the network and its research programme, and materials and references.
http://www.wits.ac.za/whp/rightsandreforms/index.htm (last accessed January 2006)

Interagency Gender Working Group (IGWG)
The IGWG is a network of NGOs, the US Agency for International Development (USAID), cooperating agencies, and the Bureau for Global Health of USAID. Its goal is to foster sustainable development and improve reproductive health and HIV/AIDS outcomes. IGWG has four priority technical areas for addressing gender equity issues and needs in the reproductive health field: gender-based violence, youth and gender, gender implications and vulnerabilities to HIV/AIDS, and male involvement. The site provides access to publications, tools and information on training and events.
http://www.igwg.org/ (last accessed January 2006)

International Centre for Reproductive Health (ICRH)
ICRH is a multidisciplinary centre operating within the Faculty of Medicine and Health Sciences at Ghent University, Belgium. In addition to research and training activities, ICRH also implements several development-related projects in Africa, Asia and Latin America. It is a WHO Collaborating Centre and provides technical assistance to national and international administrations of health and development in the fields of HIV/AIDS, STIs/STDs, family planning, mother-child health, harmful traditional practices, and sexual and gender-based violence, with focused interventions aimed at adolescents, migrants, refugees and sex workers.
http://www.icrh.org/ (last accessed January 2006)

International Planned Parenthood Federation (IPPF)
IPPF provides sexual and reproductive health services worldwide. Through its 149 Member Associations and partners, IPPF works around the world in over 180 countries, providing sexual and reproductive health information and services. IPPF works in 5 priority areas: adolescents, HIV/AIDS, abortion, access and advocacy.
http://www.ippf.org/ (last accessed January 2006)

International Women's Health Coalition (IWHC)
IWHC works in three ways to build political will and influence the policies of governments, donors, and international agencies to secure girls' and women's sexual and reproductive health and rights: by providing professional assistance and financial support, by informing

professional and public debates, and by advocacy. Its efforts focus on: youth health & rights; access to safe abortion; sexual rights and gender equality; and HIV/AIDS & women.
http://www.iwhc.org/ (last accessed January 2006)

Ipas

Ipas works globally to improve women's lives through a focus on reproductive health. It concentrates on preventing unsafe abortion, improving treatment of its complications, and reducing its consequences, striving to empower women by increasing access to services that enhance their reproductive and sexual health. The site provides access to information on Ipas' research and project work, products and publications. It includes the International Data for Evaluation of Abortion Services (IDEAS) system.
http://www.ipas.org (last accessed January 2006)

Mujer y Salud, Isis Internacional

The website presents information on their programme and documents, and includes a database on women and health with the objective of offering systematized and updated information on all aspects related to gender and health.
http://www.isis.cl/temas/salud/index.htm (last accessed January 2006)

Pacific Institute for Women's Health (PIWH)

The PIWH conducts action research, education and advocacy in the field of access to safe reproductive technology and abortion, to improve protection against STIs and HIV, and eliminate gender-based violations of human rights. Information on their international work and publications can be accessed by subject: emergency contraception, abortion access, youth, sexuality, and HIV.
http://www.piwh.org/ (last accessed January 2006)

Pathfinder International

Pathfinder International works to improve the reproductive health of women, men, and adolescents throughout the developing world with access to quality family planning information and services.
http://www.pathfind.org (last accessed January 2006)

Population Reference Bureau (PRB)

The international programmes of the USA-based PRB aim to provide timely information on population and health trends, and their implications to programme and policy communities throughout the world. The programmes work on a range of topics, including population, reproductive health, HIV/AIDS, safe motherhood, and the environment.
http://www.prb.org (last accessed January 2006)

Reproductive Health (RH) Gateway

The RH Gateway provides access to information about reproductive health on the World Wide Web. Participants include organizations that work with the Global Health Bureau of USAID. The RH Gateway is a project of the Health Information and Publications Network (HIPNet).
http://www.rhgateway.org/ (last accessed January 2006)

Reproductive Health Outlook (RHO)

This is the reproductive health website produced by the Programme for Appropriate Technology in Health (PATH). RHO is especially designed for reproductive health programme managers and decision makers working in developing countries and low-resource settings. RHO provides in-depth information on 14 reproductive health topics. Each topic includes an overview/lessons learned, key issues, an annotated bibliography, programme examples, and links.
http://www.rho.org/ (last accessed January 2006)

Right To Decide

Right To Decide is a web initiative on reproductive and sexual health and rights. It was launched during the conference 'Cairo and Beyond: Reproductive Rights and Culture' that took place in Amsterdam, the Netherlands, 7-9 March 2004. It provides an open forum for the exchange of best practices, views and news. Themes addressed include reproductive rights, youth, conflict. More themes will be added.
http://www.righttodecide.org (last accessed January 2006)

United Nations Population Fund (UNFPA)

UNFPA's work is guided by the Programme of Action adopted by 179 governments at the ICPD in 1994. UNFPA focuses on reproductive health and population issues related to the worldwide collaborative effort of meeting the Millennium Development Goals. Improving reproductive health, safe motherhood, supporting adolescents and youth, preventing HIV infection and promoting gender equality are among UNFPA's key population issues.
http://www.unfpa.org (last accessed January 2006)

gender and health: policy and practice

Women's Global Network for Reproductive Rights
The WGNRR is an autonomous network of groups and individuals in every continent who aim to achieve and support reproductive rights for women. The site contains information on WGNRR campaigns, publications and other resources.
http://www.wgnrr.nl/home.php

Sexuality

African Regional Sexuality Resources Centre (ARSRC)
The goal of the ARSRC is to promote more informed public dialogue on human sexuality and to contribute to positive changes in sexuality in Africa, by creating mechanisms for learning at the regional level. Activities under the initiative will focus on four of the most populous countries in Africa: Egypt, Kenya, Nigeria and South Africa. Action Health Incorporated, a Nigeria-based NGO, facilitates its activities and hosts the ARSRC. Training information and information resources, including the Centre's annual report, can be accessed through the website http://www.arsrc.org/ (last accessed January 2006)

Sexuality, Gender and Society in Africa programme
This is one of the current research programmes of the Nordic Africa Institute, Sweden. The website offers access to information on the programme's activities and resources.
http://www.nai.uu.se/forsk/current/sexgeneng.html (last accessed January 2006)

The South and Southeast Asia Resource Centre on Sexuality
The Centre's website hosts information on a range of issues, such as sexual and reproductive rights and health, HIV/AIDS, violence against women, and sex work. It provides information on education, training courses, electronic databases, journals, online documents, and news items related to issues of sexuality in the region. The website also hosts an online library search engine.
http://www.asiasrc.org (last accessed January 2006)

The Southeast Asian Consortium on Gender, Sexuality and Health
The Consortium was established in 2003 in recognition of the values of regional partnerships in understanding and addressing sexual health needs. Through a series of regional training courses, research and publications, the Consortium aims to promote a context-specific and gender-sensitive approach to sexuality and sexual health in research, policy advocacy and intervention in order to contribute to better sexual and reproductive health in South East Asia and China.
http://www.seaconsortium.org/ (last accessed January 2006)

Violence against women

End Violence Against Women
This website was developed to collect and share in one central location information on the latest research, tools, project reports, and communication materials produced in the worldwide struggle to end violence against women. It is designed for researchers, health communication specialists, policy makers, and others. The website provides information on the latest research, tools, publications and events related to violence against women, domestic violence and FGM.
http://www.endvaw.org/ (last accessed January 2006)

Sexual Violence Research Initiative (SVRI), WHO
The SRVI is committed to action to address gaps in research, increase interventions to prevent or respond to sexual violence, and to contribute to evaluations. The website contains documents, guidelines, links and a calendar of events.
http://www.who.int/svri/en/ (last accessed January 2006)

Toolkit for working with men and boys to prevent gender-based violence
This website, developed by the NGO Family Violence Prevention Fund, is a comprehensive toolkit designed to assist those working with men and boys to prevent gender-based violence. It provides readings, case studies, handouts, exercises, and other resources as well as community-building material.
http://toolkit.endabuse.org/Home (last accessed January 2006)

The White Ribbon Campaign (WRC): Men working to end men's violence against women
The WRC is the largest effort in the world of men working to end men's violence against women. The website includes resources and materials on how to campaign to end men's violence against women.
http://whiteribbon.com (last accessed January 2006)

About the authors

Mabel Bianco is founder and president of the Fundación para Estudio y Investigación de la Mujer (FEIM, Foundation for the Study and Investigation of Women), a research and advocacy organization based in Buenos Aires, Argentina, that has advised both government and civil society on women's sexual and reproductive health and rights since 1989. A medical doctor and epidemiologist by training, Mabel worked as a coordinator of the Women, Health and Development Programme under the Ministry of Health from 1984 to1989. She is an expert in women's health and specialist in sexual and reproductive health, and an advisor of the Pan American Health Organization (PAHO), the World Health Organization (WHO) and other United Nations organizations, as well as private international organizations. Mabel has participated in the creation of various coalitions on women's health and rights, including the National Network on Women's Health, and the Latin America and Caribbean Women's Health Network. She is a board member for Ipas and the International Women Health Coalition. She coordinates the International Women's AIDS Caucus, a group she created in 1992 as part of the International AIDS Society. She has written four books and more than 100 articles, and is a member of the editorial board of the journals Reproductive Health Matters, Sexual Health Exchange, and DeSIDAmos.

Contact address:
FEIM, Paraná 135, piso 3, dto. 13, Buenos Aires, Argentina
Tel/Fax: +54 11 4372 2763
E-mail: feim@ciudad.com.ar
Website: www.feim.org.ar

Jashodhara Dasgupta is an activist and researcher on issues of women's rights, health and gender-based violence in India. She has been involved with civil society advocacy and monitoring of women's rights especially in the field of reproductive rights and health. She works on capacity building and documentation on women's rights and gender issues at the
state level, nationally, regionally and internationally. The MacArthur Foundation has awarded her a Fellowship in Population Innovations for 1995-98. Jashodhara has been associated with research at KIT (Royal Tropical Institute), Amsterdam, the Netherlands. She is currently with SAHAYOG in India.

Contact address:
SAHAYOG, C-1485 Indira Nagar, Lucknow 226016, India
E-mail: jashodhara@sahayogindia.org

C.K. George is currently the Director of the Institute of Health Systems (IHS), Hyderabad, India. He has an academic background in medicine and public health, and coordinates multidisciplinary research and capacity building work for state and national governments, local and international NGOs and international agencies, including WHO, UN Development Programme, the British Department for International Development (DFID) and US Agency for International Development (USAID). His current research includes estimation of burden of disease and socio-economic impact of HIV;

descriptive epidemiological studies of communicable diseases and injuries; evaluation of public health programmes implemented by government and NGOs; and policy research related to financing and delivery of health care at state and national levels. He has developed and executed Masters' level academic programmes in public health and short-term training programmes related to management and delivery of primary health care. He is a member of the Health Insurance Working Group of the Insurance Regulatory Development Authority of the Government of India, and also serves in an advisory capacity to Central and State Ministries of Health. Prior to his tenure at the HIS, he has served as a primary care physician in rural areas of Kerala and was also a public health consultant to the Indian Medical Association, Kerala.

Contact address:
HIS, HACA Bhavan, Hyderabad 500 004, India
Tel.: 91-40-23210136/9; 23211013/4
Fax: 91-40-23241567
E-mail: ckgeorge@ihsnet.org.in

Anke van der Kwaak, PhD. student, is an anthropologist specialized in the field of gender and health, health systems research, and culture and health. She has worked as a researcher and trainer in the field of gender and health in Africa, particularly in the Horn of Africa. Before joining the Royal Tropical Institute (KIT), she worked for 10 years as a university lecturer at the Medical Faculty of the Free University in Amsterdam, the Netherlands. Anke has been involved in programme evaluations and gender assessments in Sudan, Somalia and Kenya. She has also conducted capacity building workshops relating to health systems research in the field of HIV/AIDS, leprosy, tuberculosis, reproductive health and female genital mutilation (FGM). Since 1988, she has participated in research, debates and discussions with respect to FGM both in the Netherlands and internationally. She has also been a co-author of a Dutch/European study on preventive and legislative measures against female circumcision in the Netherlands. Currently, Anke is a health adviser and trainer at KIT. She is also serving as project leader for an evaluation of an information, education and communication programme for Somali residents in the Netherlands.

Contact address:
Development, Policy & Practice, KIT, P.O. Box 95001, 1090 HA Amsterdam, Netherlands
Tel: +31 20 568 8497
Fax: +31 20 568 8444
E-mail: a.v.d.kwaak@kit.nl

Ireen Makwiza has a Master's degree in sociology and, as a senior social scientist, she leads the Research for Equity and Community Health Trust (REACH) HIV/AIDS research portfolio. She has conducted a number of in-depth qualitative studies on access and adherence to antiretroviral therapy (ART) in different settings in Malawi. She is also working with the WHO and the Regional Network on Equity in Health in Southern Africa (EQUINET) to facilitate a process of equity analysis in health systems in the context of ART scale up in a number of countries in Southern Africa.

Contact address:
E-mail: ireen@equi-tb-malawi.org

about the authors

Bertha Simwaka Nhlema has a Master's degree in sociology and is a senior social researcher and coordinator of REACH. She runs the Extending Services to Community (ESC) Project which involves working with store keepers, community leaders, policy makers and practitioners to enhance poor women's and men's access to TB and malaria treatment. She is currently writing up the experiences of the extent to which different social structures can be responsive to the needs of poor women and men in her PhD.

Contact address:

P.O. Box 1597, Lilongwe, Malawi

Tel./fax: +265 1 751247

E-mail: bertha@equi-tb-malawi.org

Patnice Nkhonjera is currently doing her Master's degree in theatre and development. As a social scientist at REACH, she works across the ESCP and the Linking with Civil Society (LCS) Project. Patnice has been pivotal in building and sustaining partnerships with different members of the community.

Contact address:

E-mail: pnkhonjera@equi-tb-malawi.org

Fiona Samuels has just started a new job as Research Fellow at the Overseas Development Institute (ODI), UK. Previous to that, she managed the research portfolio at the International HIV/AIDS Alliance, with a remit to develop, manage and promote research within the Alliance Secretariat, as well as with country offices and in-country partners. Here she co-ordinated a number of large-scale, multi-sited and multi-country operations research projects, focusing on HIV/AIDS related issues both within the general population and within different categories of people, including health care providers, people living with HIV/AIDS, sex workers and men who have sex with men. Fiona completed a DPhil in Social Anthropology and undertook undergraduate teaching at the University of Sussex. She has an MSc in Agricultural Economics from Oxford and a BA in Social Anthropology from the London School of Economics, UK. She has been involved in short, medium, and long-term development work for a range of NGOs, private firms and organizations, including the World Bank, DFID, the UN Children's Fund and the UN Capital Development Fund in Africa, Latin America and Asia. The work ranged from facilitating community and participatory based monitoring and evaluation, and carrying out evaluations to researching issues around social capital, stigma and discrimination, rural and urban poverty, and livelihoods. For much of the past 10 years, Fiona has been based in Zambia.

Contact address:

Research Fellow, ODI, 111 Westminster Bridge Road, London SE1 7JD, UK

E-mail: f.samuels@odi.org.uk

Lifah Sanudi has a Master' degree in sociology, and is a senior social scientist of REACH. He coordinates the LCS Project which has grown out of the success of the ESC Project. LCS involves forming partnerships with civil society, namely home-based care groups, community health committees and ex-TB patients, to enhance poor women's and men's access to TB diagnosis and treatment.

Contact address:

E-mail: lsanudi@equi-tb-malawi.org

Sehin Teferra has received a Master's degree in International Development with a focus on gender issues from Clark University in Massachusetts, USA. With a background in gender, HIV/AIDS and project implementation and monitoring, Sehin has conducted research into the relationship between gender and HIV, managed e-forums on various HIV-related topics, and is currently taking part in a baseline survey of livelihoods in southern Ethiopia. Future plans include continuing the investigation of successful strategies against FGM. An Ethiopian national, Sehin has lived in Greece, USA and Thailand.

Contact address:

E-mail: sehina2001@yahoo.com.

Sally Theobald is seconded to REACH from the Liverpool School of Tropical Medicine, UK, where she is a lecturer in Social Science & International Health. Sally has a background in gender equity, communicable diseases and health systems research. As a technical adviser, she works across all the different research projects at REACH.

Contact address:

E-mail: sjt@liv.ac.uk

Ravi K. Verma works with the Horizons Programme of the Population Council and is based in New Delhi, India. As part of his research portfolio, he designs, plans, monitors, and evaluates ongoing and innovative HIV/AIDS operations research projects, in close collaboration with local partners in India and other countries in the region. His current projects include: addressing gender norms and masculinity as a strategy to reduce HIV risk behaviours among young men from low income communities in Mumbai; building social capital among marginalized but key population for HIV prevention; and understanding the context and dynamics of same sex behaviour among truckers. He serves in an advisory capacity to the International AIDS Vaccine Initiative in India and other national level bodies, and maintains strategic partnerships with donor, government and NGO partners. Prior to joining the Population Council, he was on the faculty of the International Institute for Population Sciences (IIPS), Mumbai. At IIPS for over two decades, he managed multi-faceted collaborative demographic studies, sexual health intervention research projects, and conducted national studies on fertility, family planning and reproductive health and sexual behaviours; designed and executed international courses and training programmes; delivered sustained technical assistance to public sector institutions and NGOs in reproductive health and HIV/AIDS; and developed and managed multidisciplinary teams. He has published extensively in both national and international journals, and more recently co-edited a book on sexuality in the times of AIDS in the Indian context.

Contact address:

Population Council/Horizons Programme, 53 Lodhi Estate, New Delhi 110003, India
Tel: 91-11-24610193
E-mail: raviverma@pcindia.org

Madeleen Wegelin-Schuringa is a social scientist with 26 years' experience working on: slum improvement, sanitation, water, hygiene, community mobilization and HIV/AIDS. She has expertise in project planning and implementation, strategy development, monitoring and evaluation, and training. She has an international reputation as a facilitator of multistakeholder participation. She has worked with multilateral organizations (UN Educational, Scientific and Cultural Organization, World Bank, UN Centre for Human Settlements, UNAIDS), bilateral government organizations (DGIS Netherlands, Ireland Aid, DFID) and international and local NGOs. Her understanding of the way these organizations function enables her to work at national level and at local level (district and community), and to bridge the gap between these levels. She has lived and worked for 12 years in Asia (Pakistan,

Thailand, Philippines, Indonesia) and 3 years in Africa (Kenya), and has worked on short-term assignments in many countries of Asia and Africa. At present, Madeleen is working as a senior AIDS adviser at KIT. She managed the development of a toolkit for local responses to HIV/AIDS for UNAIDS. In addition, she is involved in strategy development for mainstreaming HIV/AIDS in different development sectors, and in capacity building for this at different levels (district, national, international).

Contact address:

Development, Policy & Practice, KIT, P.O. Box 95001, 1090 HA Amsterdam, Netherlands

Tel: +31 20 5688332

Fax: +31 20 5688444

E-mail: m.wegelin@kit.nl

Miriam Zoll is a writer, and a researcher and analyst for the UN and other international public policy institutions. In 2005, she was awarded a Research Fellowship at the Massachusetts Institute of Technology's (MIT) Centre for International Studies' Programme on Human Rights and Justice. Focusing on HIV/AIDS in sub-Saharan Africa, her research addresses how the enforcement of women's economic rights, particularly compensation for unpaid HIV/AIDS sector labour, should be used as a job creation strategy to alleviate poverty and improve care and support for millions of orphans and vulnerable children. Working with the UN system since 1999, she has written and edited numerous reports and publications. In 2004-2005, she was a lead analyst and writer for an unprecedented 17-country USAID/UNICEF/UNAIDS/World Food Programme-Futures Group International initiative assessing multiple aspects of orphan policies and programmes in sub-Saharan Africa. To view the country documents, please go to www.futuresgroup.com/ovc. At the Beijing Plus Five Review Conference in 2000, she launched UNIFEM's historic biennial publication, Progress of the world's women. In 2003-2004, she was the lead global researcher and editorial consultant for a Joint UN Agency publication on Women and HIV/AIDS: confronting the crisis.

Contact address:

E-mail: zollm@mit.edu

Sarah Cummings, **Henk van Dam** and **Minke Valk** are information specialists within the Information & Library Services (ILS) of KIT. They are editors of the Gender, Society & Development series. Sarah, Henk and Minke are also involved in the production of thematic web resources called Specials.

Contact address:

ILS, KIT, P.O. Box 95001, 1090 HA Amsterdam, Netherlands

Tel: +31 20 568 8594/8573/8347/8344

Fax: +31 20 6654 423

E-mail: s.cummings@kit.nl; h.v.dam@kit.nl; m.valk@kit.nl

Website: www.kit.nl/ils/html/gender_society_development.asp